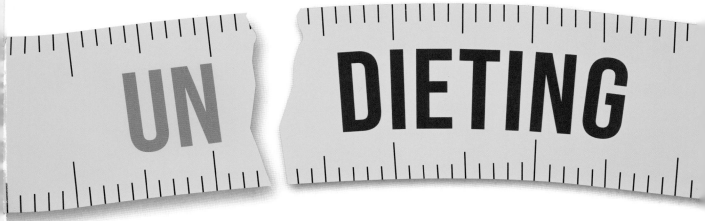

UN DIETING

Freedom from the
Bewildering World of Fad Diets

LISA KILGOUR, CHN

Fountaindale Public Library
Bolingbrook, IL
(630) 759-2102

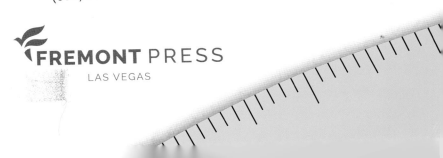

FREMONT PRESS

LAS VEGAS

First published in 2020 by Fremont Press

Copyright © 2020 Lisa Kilgour

All rights reserved

No part of this publication may be reproduced or distributed in any form or by any means, electronic or mechanical, or stored in a database or retrieval system, without prior written permission from the publisher.

ISBN-13: 978-1-628604-10-8

The information included in this book is for educational purposes only. It is not intended or implied to be a substitute for professional medical advice. The reader should always consult his or her healthcare provider to determine the appropriateness of the information for his or her own situation or if he or she has any questions regarding a medical condition or treatment plan. Reading the information in this book does not constitute a physician-patient relationship. The statements in this book have not been evaluated by the Food and Drug Administration. The products or supplements in this book are not intended to diagnose, treat, cure, or prevent any disease. The author and publisher expressly disclaim responsibility for any adverse effects that may result from the use or application of the information contained in this book.

Author photos by Kodiak BC

Cover design by Charisse Reyes

Interior design by Elita San Juan, Allan Santos & Crizalie Olimpo

Printed in Canada

TC 0120

TABLE OF CONTENTS

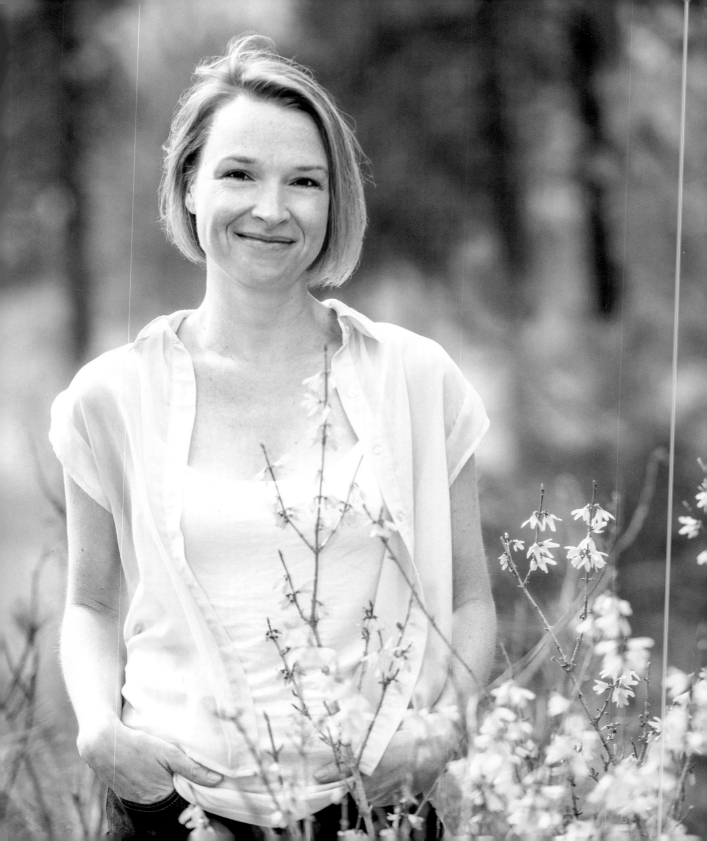

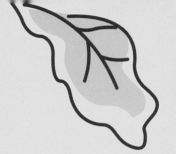

To the readers—the brave people who are ready to leave dieting culture behind, listen to their bodies, and become their own nutrition experts.

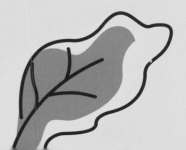

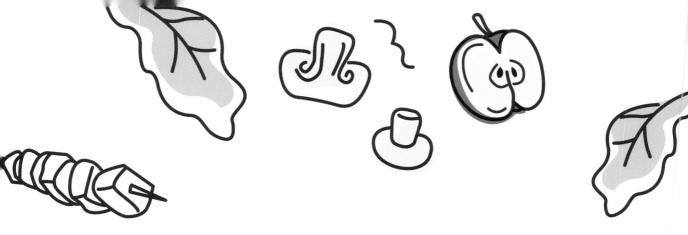

INTRODUCTION

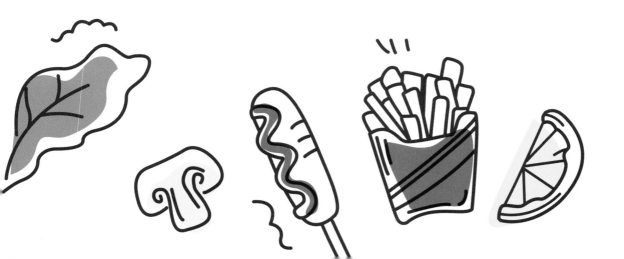

My journey toward holistic nutrition wasn't exactly straight-forward. I didn't grow up on an organic farm, and I didn't love Brussels sprouts when I was a kid. In all honesty, I thought broccoli tasted like dirt until I was in my mid-twenties.

I first learned about nutrition so I could help myself feel better. I was desperately in need of assistance, and I didn't know where to turn, so I dove in and learned for myself. I slowly transitioned my highly processed diet of sweetened peanut butter, sugary cereal, and little else to a healthy whole-food diet. Because of my experience, I deeply understand that a big dietary change is possible, but it's best done slowly. For me, it happened at a snail's pace.

My journey to health started in the summer of 2002 when a company that makes a whole-food supplement hired me. I don't know why they hired me: Two nutritionists were my competition for the job, and I knew absolutely *nothing* about nutrition. Zero, zilch, nada. And I'm sure I didn't win the hiring team over with my gray complexion and the dark circles under my eyes, but they took a chance with me. I'm still so grateful for that job; it changed my life.

I didn't find the courage to try the company's signature product until I'd been working there for a few weeks. The supplement was very green—it even *tasted* very green. It was full of grasses and algae, which 2002 Lisa found very unappetizing. One day, I decided to give it a chance and gulped it down. It wasn't *terrible*, but I was far from sold on it. Each morning, I plugged my nose and drained my green and grassy cup, hoping for the best. About two weeks later, I woke up one morning feeling...different.

To help you understand how different I felt that morning, I need to tell you a bit about how awful I'd felt just one day earlier. The descent into my terrible state had started when I first left home to go to university.

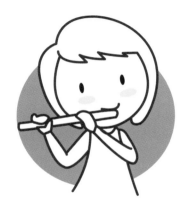

My first year in university was pretty darn wonderful. It was 1997, and I had gotten into a competitive performance music program to study the flute. I was thrilled to be there. The program was filled with people who were just like me—those who felt music deeply and understood the language of music in the same way as I did. Music was the vehicle through which I could feel and express emotions, and I had found my tribe of like-minded musical people. I even got to play and record with my all-time favorite rock band, The Rheostatics. Life was pretty magical.

The Dark Clouds Gather

It was in my second year of university that the trouble began. The apartment I had lined up before I went home for summer vacation fell through just two weeks before classes started. Finding a different affordable place to live in a city with less than 1 percent vacancy was almost impossible. As the school year started, some very kind friends let me sleep on their couch, but I was still under a ton of stress. I spent almost two months continually searching before I found a decent place to live—well, decent if I ignored the giant jumping, biting cockroaches. Unfortunately, the daily apartment search had cut into my studies, and I was falling behind fast.

Just after I got settled into my new place, I was asked to play in the pit orchestra for the musical *My Fair Lady*. It was a community theater production, and it was a bit of a slog—seven shows in six days, with each show clocking in at more than four hours. All of the stress on top of my terrible student diet had triggered a severe injury. By the end of the run, I had shooting pain down my arms, and I had severe tendinitis in my thumbs. My first real "gig" created my first significant injury—one that almost ended my musical education.

Through lots and lots of physical therapy, my arms and thumbs healed, but the inflammation continued. I developed asthma the next year, and by my final year of school, I was deeply exhausted. I could barely get through each day. As time went on, I felt worse and worse. My thinking was so foggy that I frequently forgot what day of the week it was and where I was going. I got lost in the subway system many times because I had gotten on the wrong subway car or gotten off at the wrong stop, thinking it was Thursday instead of Wednesday. I had forgotten what it felt like to feel good. I had no memory of what it felt like to wake up and be excited for the day or to read something and feel like I was retaining it. I didn't miss my old life because, frankly, I couldn't remember it. I knew something was wrong with me, but countless doctors and specialists told me that I was just fine.

Today, I can look back and better understand what was going on. My eating habits were the primary culprit. A steady diet of sugary cereal, white bread, sweetened peanut butter, and packaged meals was highly inflammatory and taking a negative toll. My body and mind were *starving* for nutrients. What

I find interesting now is that not one of the many doctors I visited during that time asked me about my diet or the stress in my life. By the spring of 2002 I was sick and tired of feeling sick and tired, and that's when I decided it was time to do my own investigation.

The Sun Started Shining Again

Then that day in the summer of 2002, after I had replenished my body with enough nutrients, I suddenly woke up feeling different. I felt...clear. The fog had lifted, and my mind felt sharp again. I suddenly remembered that I liked to learn, and I liked to read. I will *never* forget that moment; it was when I got my life back.

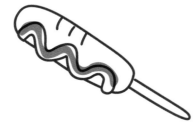

After realizing the difference that adding just one whole food made to my mental and physical health, it became my obsession to learn more about health and nutrition. I spent hours every day reading and learning. I couldn't get enough! I worked in customer service at the whole-food supplement company, and my job allowed me to speak with tons of people every day and learn constantly. This is where I developed my love of helping people. The summer of 2002 was a pivotal moment in my life.

A few years later, I went back to school with my new, sharp mind to learn more about nutrition. Once again, I was with a group of like-minded people, but this time I had the energy and focus to make the most of it. In 2007, I graduated at the top of my class, something that would have been impossible just a few short years earlier.

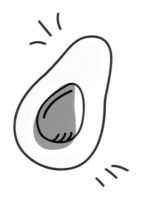

It took me about six years to slowly shift my diet from the highly inflammatory and processed diet of my university years to the diet I have now. That may seem like a long time, but it was the amount of time that I needed to make a *big* dietary change. I went from barely eating any fruit or vegetables to enjoying a diet filled to the brim with them (and I really like them!). Because I took things slowly, I never "fell off" these changes. Well, there was one time I fell off because I tried an extreme diet shift.

The Myth of a Quick Fix

I had been dealing with some immune system issues, and I was curious to see if a raw-food diet could rebalance my system. Years of antibiotics and sugary foods had left my gut bacteria in a sorry state, and I was hopeful that a raw diet would "fix" it.

I don't have a lot of willpower when it comes to dietary changes, which is why I usually take things so slowly. I need to make things as easy as possible so I can be successful. But this time, I was really motivated to tackle the immune challenges and ready to make a dramatic change.

I decided to be kind to myself and start with a trial of just one weekend. Just two days of all raw food. On my way home from work on Friday night, I picked up all of my favorite raw foods, including lots of fruit to satisfy my sugar cravings. I was all set!

The next morning, I woke up excited to have my raw breakfast. It was strawberries, and I love strawberries, but they really weren't satisfying that morning. By lunchtime, I had eaten everything I had bought the night before, trying to fill myself up. Nothing worked. I had to leave for a hair appointment in the afternoon, and even though I was all bundled up, the winter cold chilled me to the bone.

By the end of my hair appointment, I was at the end of my rope. I was so hungry and so cold that I was desperate for something warm. On my way home, I picked up an order from a fast food joint, and so ended my attempt at a raw diet.

You might think that I should have stuck it out longer to let my body adjust to the new way of eating or that I didn't have enough willpower to drive through the inevitable hard part. I see it differently, though. That feeling that I was starving and the fact that no amount of raw food was satiating were signs that I wasn't feeding my body the food it needed. Maybe if I had chosen a weekend during the summer, when all of those raw foods were in season, my body would have reacted differently. Maybe if I had chosen to make healthy and warm foods, I would have had a completely different reaction. All I know is that my body wasn't having it.

This may seem like an extreme example of a diet not working, but I've seen a version of it with every client on a restrictive diet or cleanse over the years. They may be able to follow it for weeks or even months before their fast food or chocolate cake moment, but it always happens.

I deprived my body for only six hours, so my fast food indulgence was satisfied with just one meal. I've noticed a pattern among my clients who have much more willpower than I do: The longer they say no to a food, the longer their food indulgence detour when they fall off the wagon. Many clients who have spent six months or more on a restrictive diet might spend many months (sometimes years) inside a continuous period of indulgence in everything that they'd denied themselves during the diet period.

The Kinder Way

This conundrum is why diets don't work. Depriving yourself of food you love or need doesn't work. Also, I believe that willpower can be a harmful tool in a health journey. It lets you ignore your body's signals as you work to stay on whatever diet plan you've committed to. I feel that my lack of willpower is my superpower; my body always needs to be on board with any changes I make; when it is, the changes come easily and are permanent.

Undieting is a much kinder way to treat yourself. It's a practice of tapping into your body's innate wisdom. Your body wants to be healthy and balanced, and it already knows exactly what it needs each day. By learning how to listen to your body, you quickly learn how to interpret your body's signals as they guide you to your uniquely healthy way of eating.

In my private practice as a nutritionist, I've worked with thousands of people, and I've seen the power of undieting over and over again. By focusing on whole foods and learning your body's unique language, you can gain tons of energy, feel fantastic, and balance your weight—all without counting calories, weighing your food, and denying yourself.

Today, the marketing for each new diet proclaims that it's the perfect diet and the solution to everyone's problems, but when you follow a set diet or meal plan, you're negating your body's needs and depriving yourself of food that you love.

You don't need to say no to *everything* you enjoy just to eat a healthy diet. Instead, when you tap in and listen to what your body is looking for, when you understand your body's language, you can create real health—energy, clear thinking, and pleasure. Pleasurable food *can* be a part of a healthy diet.

When I look back at the exhausted and foggy version of myself from 2002, I can see that making any major dietary change would have been impossible. It's so hard to try anything new while you're absolutely bone tired. But you don't have to make a huge change. Your body starts the healing process with each change you make, no matter how small. You could start with just one healthy meal or a piece of fruit in the afternoon. The fact that my body lit up and cleared out the fog a few weeks after I made one teeny tiny change wasn't an anomaly. I've seen it repeated hundreds of times.

The principles of undieting can work in your life. Small, simple changes are powerful. And, the best part is that they're permanent. Say good-bye to fad dieting and hello to real-life healthy eating!

I've divided this book into three parts. In Part 1, I take you on a deep dive into nutrition and what to look for when choosing healthy food. In Part 2, I unpack dieting culture. I discuss how politics, lobbyists, and poor science contributed to a culture where new fad dieting ideas and increasingly unrealistic norms of physical appearance bombard us almost every day.

In Part 3, I take you through the steps to become your own nutrition expert. I explain how to uncover your body's language by listening to your cravings and your digestive system and paying attention to what feels right to you.

As you read, you'll quickly notice a central theme in this book: Your body always wins. It already knows exactly how you need fuel it to feel your best; you just have to uncover that need. By undieting, you'll dissolve any guilt and confusion you might feel while bringing joy and pleasure back into each of your meals.

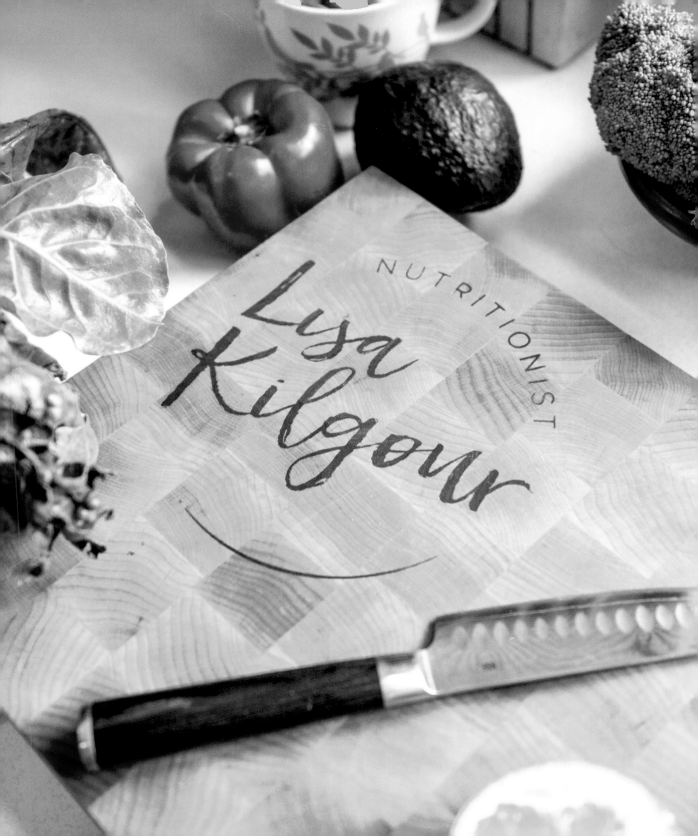

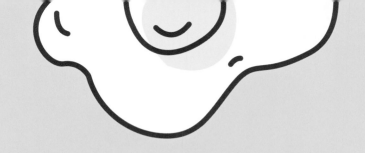

PART 1

NUTRITION PRINCIPLES

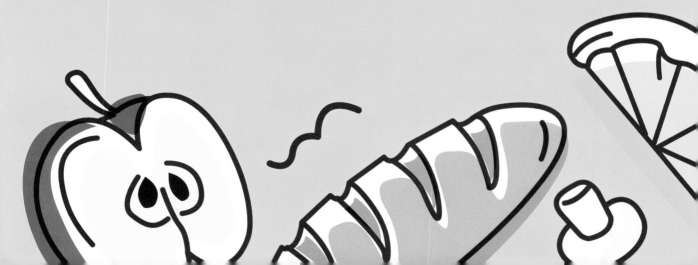

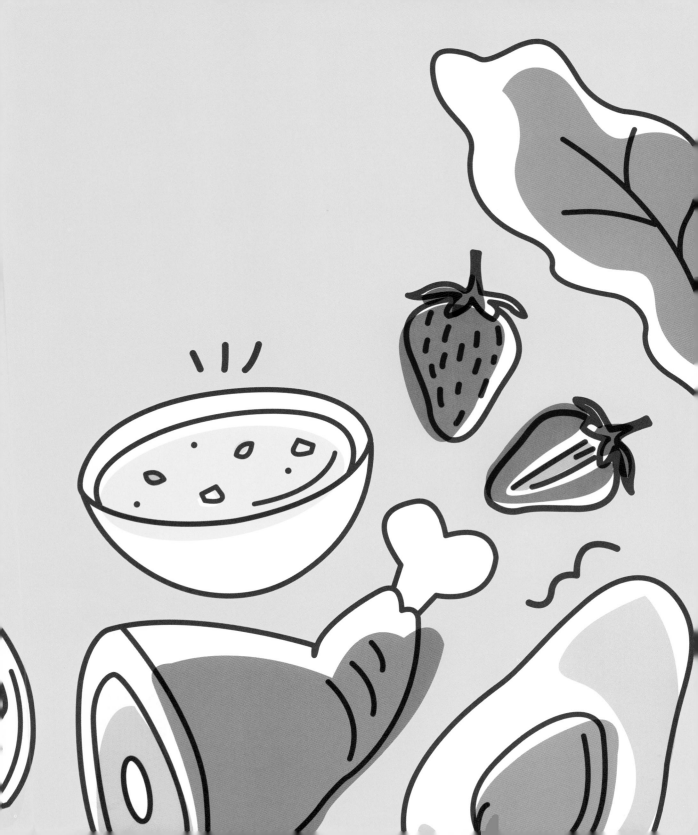

chapter
01

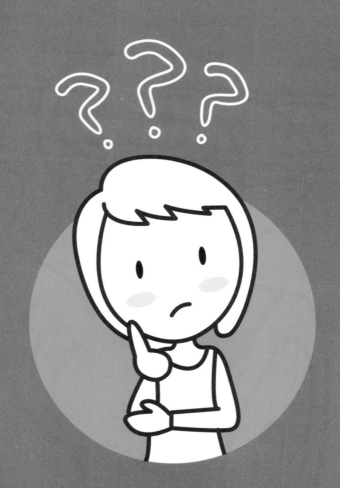

THE NUTS AND BOLTS OF NUTRITION

With so many experts touting the latest and greatest diet programs, most of which vilify one nutrient or the other, many people struggle to figure out which nutrition concept or way of eating is right for them. Is vegan best? Or Paleo? What about a raw food diet? Or maybe the ketogenic diet is the way to go?

This confusion has moved people away from attending to the body's natural cues. Many people struggle to understand their body's unique balance of carbs, fats, and proteins. When you follow a trendy diet, you ignore your body's signals, which can bring about feelings of deprivation, frustration, and guilt. It's impossible to stay on any sort of diet or meal plan forever, so eventually, you're going to "fall off the wagon." Sadly, that often leads to more confusion and possibly nutrient deprivation than when you started.

You can walk away from this confusion by learning to tune back into your body and find exactly how it wants you to feed it each day. No more counting, no more questioning, and no more feeling deprived of your favorite food. The subject of this book, undieting, is all about food freedom, and that feels fantastic.

In the grand scheme of things, the question "What should I eat?" is a relatively new concept for humans. Not very long ago—just a generation or two—people knew what to eat; they simply ate what was available. People ate the food that was grown and produced closest to them, and they prepared it in traditional ways.

In North America and most of Europe, people ate lots of fresh fruit and veggies all summer and fall and switched to canned fruit, apples, pears, and root veggies (the foods that they could easily store in a root cellar) all winter. The diet was lighter in summer and heavier in the winter when people needed to stay warm. There was no calorie counting, and rarely did anyone think about whether they'd eaten too many carbs or too little protein. Animal fat was considered a precious commodity and always was saved in jars for later use. People ate with the seasons as nature intended, so no one ever ate salads and strawberries in January because those foods weren't available.

Are people healthier today than two generations ago? When it comes to preventable diet-related diseases like heart disease, diabetes, and obesity, the answer is no.

Let's Talk About Macros

In the last few decades, nutrition experts have been spouting a different idea or theory just about every day, and one particular question among people following these trends has become common: "What are my macros?"

Macros are the three main nutritional components that humans need to survive—carbohydrates, fat, and protein. If you don't get enough of each macro, you can feel tired, unfueled, and unbalanced. When people ask what their specific macros are, they're asking what balance of carbohydrates, fat, and protein is the "right" combination, as if there is one combination that will work for 7.5 billion different humans.

This idea of balancing carbs, fat, and protein is a concept that comes out of flawed nutritional science and profit-driven food manufacturing. Nutritional science keeps looking for a perfect ratio (spoiler: no one has found it yet and probably won't), and food manufacturers like to jump on each popular fad (sugar free, fat free, reduced fat, etc.) to create the hottest new products. So far, none of the suggested combinations has been rigorously tested and determined to be the "perfect" balance.

So, experts keep proposing different opinions—way too many to count. Today, protein is king, and many nutrition and fitness experts are preaching a balance of 40 percent protein, 30 percent fat, 30 percent carbohydrate. Some more extreme fitness trainers have recommended an extremely high-protein diet of 60 percent protein, 20 percent fat, 20 percent carbohydrate (yikes!). The latest popular diet—the ketogenic diet—says that fat is the real nutritional king, and the balance should be 70 percent fat, 20 percent protein, and 10 percent carbohydrate. However, not too long ago (just ten years or so), the "perfect balance" was supposed to be 60 percent carbohydrate, 20 percent protein, and 20 percent fat. I can hear all of the current high-fat and high-protein promoters crying out "NO!" to that combination.

You can see the problem with profit-driven fads. These diets may feel like they're effective, for a little while anyway, but they rarely work well in the long term. Very few people have continued health benefits (weight loss, increased energy, etc.) for any length of time after following a fad diet. Instead, listen to your body to determine your nutritional ratios rather than concerning yourself with the latest get-slim-quick scheme.

If you look at traditional diets—those that have kept humans healthy for generations—you see every different kind of combination of nutrients you can imagine. You'll find extremes from the heavy meat and blood diet of the Masai people to the high-starch diet throughout South America and South Asia. No one is ever going to find the "perfect balance" of macros for all human beings because everyone is different. Your body already knows exactly what it wants; you just need to learn to listen and uncover what it's looking for.

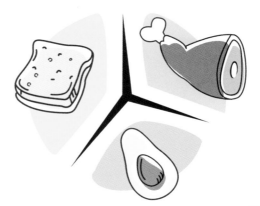

Macros Expanded

Let's start by getting a sense of what all of these crazy macros are and what they do in your body. This way, you'll have a better understanding of why your body may be craving (or asking for) different foods.

CARBOHYDRATES

I'm starting with carbohydrates because this nutrient is so very important, and people seem to have forgotten how precious and vital carbs are. (Read Chapter 5 for more about the history of the vilification of carbohydrates.)

Until relatively recently, carbs wore the golden halo that protein wears now. For many decades, carbohydrates were seen as the most important macronutrient. Why? Because you need a steady supply of glucose in your bloodstream to move and think and do everything you need to do in your day. Fruits, veggies, beans, and whole grains are sources of glucose. They're also full of fiber, which is important for the trillion microbes that live in your gut. In this section, I explain this currently undervalued macronutrient, and I hope you start to understand why the heck you're craving carbs all day! (It's 'cause you need them.)

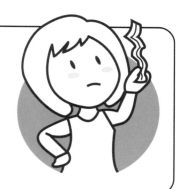

KETOGENIC DIET

The ketogenic diet has shown that the body can use ketones instead of glucose for energy, but the jury is still out on the sustainability and the health implications of this diet. I prefer to stick to the method the human body has perfected over time, which is burning glucose and using ketones only when there's no glucose available. Call me crazy, but I think the human body is pretty amazing, and you don't need to hijack your body's preferences.

Carbohydrates are a combination of monosaccharides (single sugars), oligosaccharides (short chains of sugars), polysaccharides (long chains of sugars), and fiber. All unrefined carbohydrate foods are chock-full of vitamins, minerals, antioxidants, and polyphenols.

Your body digests chains of sugars and turns them into fuel. Right now, as you read this sentence, your brain is using glucose to process your thoughts, and your muscles are using glucose to hold up your book or e-reader. Your body needs a steady trickle of glucose throughout the day.

Foods with longer chains of sugar and more fiber digest slowly and provide the slowest trickle of glucose. Single sugars, which are in fruit, honey, and refined sugary foods, provide a faster hit of glucose and energy, which can be useful when you need it, but it's a problem if your blood sugar spikes too high. When you need an extra boost of energy, fruit provides the perfect burst of sweetness. It's perfectly packaged to provide just enough glucose to bring your blood sugar up but not so much that it causes a blood sugar spike. Plus, fruit comes with some fiber to slow down the sugar hit, and it's full of lots of energy-enhancing vitamins. Otherwise, it's best to focus on whole food sources of carbohydrates that provide those slow-burning long chains of sugar, like beans and veggies.

Recently, I've heard this question about starchy foods a lot: "Doesn't it just turn into sugar?" People who ask that are usually talking about healthy whole-food starchy vegetables like potatoes because they've heard that those foods convert to glucose just as white sugar does.

The answer is yes; starchy foods do eventually turn into sugar. But this statement overlooks the fact that this can be said of more than just starchy foods. All carbs turn into sugar (including nonstarchy veggies like broccoli), and that's not a bad thing. What matters is how quickly your body digests the food and breaks down the sugar chains. Those things determine how much glucose is in your bloodstream at each moment. What you want is a trickle of glucose or sugar from healthy whole-food starchy vegetables and grains, not the spike in glucose from refined white sugar.

Carbs and Water Weight

If you've ever followed a low-carb diet for a few days, then you've witnessed the phenomenon of immediate weight loss— like, pounds and pounds of weight just falling off your body. It seems magical, and it's what the low-carb diet promoters count on to inspire you to continue the diet. There's nothing like immediate results to keep you on board.

But, I'm sorry to say, you hadn't lost actual pounds of fat—that's physiologically impossible. You'd lost water weight, and you'd probably become a bit dehydrated. Anytime you lose or gain pounds overnight, you've just lost or gained some water weight. And it can be a lot! I've gained and lost more than 8 pounds of water in a single day!

Carbohydrates bind to water. The more carbs you eat, the more water you'll hold onto. Keep this in mind the next time you enjoy something sweet. It didn't immediately "go to your hips"; you've just (temporarily) gained some water weight.

The Benefit of Starches

Traditionally, humans have eaten a pile of starchy foods— lots and lots of potatoes, sweet potatoes, root veggies, and squashes. Today, there are still many traditional cultures that eat a lot of starches, and they're healthy for it.

Starchy foods are full of slow-burning sugar chains and fiber. This combo slows down the digestion of the sugars, so you get a nice little trickle of glucose for hours. The indigestible fiber also feeds the good bacteria in your gut, which research is finding can help rev up your metabolism and balance your immune system. It also helps your body handle sugars.

Without a steady source of dietary fiber, your elimination pathway slows down (that's a polite way of saying you won't poop as well), and your gut bacteria can starve. Researchers have connected low numbers and low diversity in gut bacteria to chronic inflammation and obesity. So, keep munching on those fibrous starchy foods!

Vitamin, Mineral, and Antioxidant Abundance

Scientists have found that a nutrient-rich diet, which is filled to the brim with vitamins, minerals, and antioxidants, is the healthiest. The best source for all of these nutrients is carb-laden foods like veggies, fruit, whole grains, and beans. You can become nutrient-deficient either by eating too many refined foods or by shunning carbs and starches in a low-carb diet.

The manufacturing process for refined sugar and flour removes all of these amazing nutrients. Furthermore, your body needs B vitamins, magnesium, and chromium to assimilate and use the energy from sugary foods, but you can't digest refined foods unless they steal these nutrients from your body. Manufacturers add some of these nutrients back to enriched white flour, but those added nutrients aren't a substitute for the real ones that were removed.

Over time, eating refined foods can lead to many deficiencies, which can lead to exhaustion, tight and sore muscles, and blood sugar irregularities. Plus, your body will keep craving these processed foods because it's looking for the nutrients it could get from their whole-food cousins.

The Reasons Behind Cutting Carbs

There are a few reasons that low-carb diets have been so popular for the last decade or so. One reason is that some researchers have connected carbs to weight gain, high blood sugar, and inflammation. Sure sounds like a reason to cut them out of your diet, right? Well, it's not quite that simple.

Remember that steady trickle of glucose you need in your bloodstream to keep your motor running all day? Anytime you have glucose in your bloodstream, your pancreas releases an equal amount of insulin. Insulin plays a role as a gatekeeper for your cells. Your cells want and need glucose, but too much can be a problem, so your body uses insulin to make sure just the right amount of glucose gets into your cells.

On every cell is an insulin receptor, and insulin fits that receptor like a key to a lock. When the cell asks for some glucose, insulin unlocks the cell to allow a bit of glucose to get in. The problem starts when you eat something like a sugary treat: you get a burst of glucose instead of a trickle. First, you get a boost of insulin to help get some of that glucose into your hungry cells, but if your insulin level is too high, then it signals your body that you have more energy than you need.

Your miraculous body saves that extra energy for later; first, your body stores the energy in your liver and muscles. If those storage spots are full, then your body stores the excess energy in your fat cells. Over time, if you have too many glucose bursts, your body has more and more extra energy, and you start to gain weight. It's not one sweet treat that causes weight gain but daily bursts over some time.

Carbs can be "fattening," but this blanket statement has some flaws, just like the low-fat rhetoric in the 1980s did. If you eat fewer carbs, your blood sugar may be steadier, and you'll avoid weight gain and high blood sugar. But for many, reducing carbs comes at a price. First, it can lead to deprivation and cravings. Over time, a low-carb diet, especially if you're active, can lead to lower thyroid function (which leads to a slower metabolism), higher cortisol (a stress hormone), depressed mood, and muscle loss.

You don't need to avoid *all* carbs to lose weight; you just need to avoid refined sugars and flours that are full of fast-digesting sugars without any fiber.

This is key, so I'm going to repeat it: You don't need to avoid all carbs—just the refined ones. Unfortunately, whole grains and starchy veggies have been put in the "bad" category. Let's pull them outta there and get them back onto your plate!

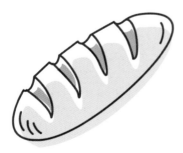

Don't Drink Sugar

Sweetened drinks like soda, sugary coffees, and pasteurized juices are particularly hard on your body. Because the beverages don't include any fiber or anything else to digest, the sugar in them hits your bloodstream quickly, causing a great big burst of glucose. The trouble is that when you drink something sweet, without having anything to chew or digest, your body doesn't even register that you've eaten anything! Consequently, your body still thinks you're hungry and keeps asking for more food. Sugary drinks aren't found in nature, so your body struggles to understand where all of the glucose in them comes from.

So, please, just don't drink sugary drinks. Full stop.

Carbohydrate Deficiency

Some bodies thrive on a lower-carb diet. If you have lots of energy, think clearly, and feel great on a low-carb diet, then you've found a way of eating that's excellent for you. However, some people need to eat starchy food regularly to stoke their internal fires.

Symptoms that your body is asking for more healthy starchy food are cravings for sweets or starches, low mood, sluggishness, and muscle loss. (Your muscles need carbs too!)

Women tend to be extra sensitive to a low-carb diet and can also feel hormonal imbalances after reducing carbs. Even if women eat enough calories, a low-carb diet can stop their periods in the same way starvation can. A low-carb diet can cause fertility issues, disrupted sleep, and weight gain around the middle. Low-carb diets can affect men as well; research has shown that men who exercise but don't eat enough carbs have higher cortisol and lower testosterone levels.

Cutting carbs when your body wants and needs them can cause a cycle of deprivation and bingeing. You can say no for a few days, weeks, or months, but eventually, your body forces you to get what it wants. It's not a sign you don't have enough willpower; it's a sign that your body is desperate for a steady supply of energy! Add some healthy, high-fiber, carby whole foods to your diet, and you'll find that your body feels a lot more balanced.

FAT, FAT, GLORIOUS FAT

Fat is currently on deck to make a major comeback. The low-fat 1980s are long gone, and in the last few years, there's been a huge surge in high-fat fad diets.

Despite years of "fat is good" media attention, in my experience, I find that most folks are still low-fat eaters. Over the years I've been in practice, I've found that fat is still the main macronutrient people are deficient in.

This deficiency isn't surprising, though. The low-fat diet craze lasted almost two decades! That was enough time for most people to forget to pay attention to fat. Although you may not actively shun it, you're probably not actively adding it either, as you might with protein.

Signs of having an overall deficiency in dietary fat exhibit as dryness (dry skin, eyes, hair, sinuses) and an imbalance in your immune system. Fat also plays an important role in inflammation in your body. If your skin is dry or you're dealing with chronic inflammation, then you might be deficient in fat.

The low-fat craze also sparked the use of many problematic highly processed fats like margarine, trans fat, and refined vegetable oils. Trans fat has now taken its rightful place as a villainous fat, but highly processed fats and oils, like vegetable oil and highly refined canola oil, still have a golden halo. In this section, I explain fat's role in the body and how to tell a "good" fat from a "bad" one.

Why Fat Was Vilified in the 1980s

In the late 1970s and early 1980s, the experts said people should reduce fat in their diets for weight loss because fat is more calorie-dense than protein and carbs. Fat has 9 calories per gram versus protein and carbohydrates, which have 4 calories per gram. The thought was that reducing dietary fat would mean eating fewer calories. And, if you eat fewer calories, then you'll lose weight, right?

Unfortunately, no. The U.S. and Canadian governments announced low-fat recommendations in 1977, and the UK and Australian governments followed suit in 1980. Since that time, there's been a staggering increase in obesity and heart disease in those countries.

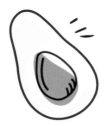

But how could this be? How could people have gained weight when they were eating less fat?

The simple answer is this: Fat is satiating. Fat has been such an important part of human evolution that your body only feels full once it's had enough fat. Early on, human beings developed large, fatty brains that needed a steady supply of dietary fat, and humans' bodies still need fat to power their brains. Fat in the stomach sends a signal to the brain as a signal of satiety, and studies have found that people eat more calories when they're on a low-fat diet because the brain isn't getting the signal it needs. Fat also slows down the digestion of simple sugars, which keeps your blood sugar down and helps you stay full for a lot longer.

Fat Is a Carrier

Let me tell you a little-known fact about healthy eating: Adding butter, coconut oil, or a healthy oil to your veggies is a good thing. Your salad needs an oil-and-vinegar dressing, and your sweet potatoes could use some butter.

Fat is a carrier for critical nutrients. Vitamins A, D, E, and K are fat-soluble, which means they need fat to be digested and absorbed. Some foods also include fat-soluble phytonutrients and antioxidants like lycopene and beta carotene. Beta carotene, otherwise known as pro-vitamin A, needs fat to be absorbed and converted into vitamin A. So, your lycopene-rich tomatoes need a boost from some extra-virgin olive oil, and your beta carotene–rich carrots, squash, and sweet potatoes are crying out for a bit of organic butter to help your body make use of the antioxidants.

Fat Is So Important in the Body

Your body uses dietary fats in so many ways that there's rarely any excess to be stored or even burned as energy. For example, your body uses fat to manufacture hormones and create cell membranes, and it's a major part of your brain and nervous system. Your brain is 60 percent fat!

Dietary fat very rarely becomes fat in your body; it's (almost) physiologically impossible. You store the energy from dietary fat only after your body has used it for all of its functions in the body, like making cell walls, hormones, brain tissue, prostaglandins, neurotransmitters, and aiding in the absorption and of those vitamins I talked about earlier. After all this, your body burns fat as fuel only after it has used all of the glucose.

If the high-fat diet craze has taught people anything, it's that you can consume large amounts of fat and still lose weight. So, please add more healthy fat into your diet, and don't worry; you won't be adding any extra padding around your middle.

Fat Is Nutrient Poor

It might seem counterintuitive that although I'm a *huge* fat lover and promoter, I'm not a fan of a super high-fat diet (like the 60 to 80 percent fat ketogenic diet). Fat is *mega* important to the body, but it's also nutrient-poor. Dietary fat lacks in vitamins, minerals, and many antioxidants. Over time, a very high-fat diet can result in many nutrient deficiencies, which is the reason balancing all macronutrients is key.

Types of Dietary Fat

When people moved away from the fat phobia of the 1980s and 1990s, certain types of fat, like unsaturated fat, were quickly embraced and hailed as healthy by many experts. But, a particularly important type of fat, saturated fat, is still waiting on the sidelines for its time in the spotlight.

I'd like to invite you to look at fat a little differently. You'll quickly see in this section how valuable all types of fat are (especially saturated fat), but quality matters. How a fat is processed and stored is what determines how healthy it is; its type isn't a determining factor. Fat is very intolerant to industrial processing, so fats that are as close to natural as possible are always the best.

An important note: All fatty foods are a combination of different types of fats. No fat is *all* saturated or unsaturated, but each fat is classified into one category based on which is the dominant type. Butter is usually considered to be 100 percent saturated fat, but it is only 51 percent saturated and contains many other types of fat, including polyunsaturated fats. Even extra-virgin olive oil, which is categorized as a super healthy monounsaturated fat, is 14 percent saturated.

Saturated Fat

Saturated fats are commonly found in animal-based foods, as well as in coconut oil and palm oil. Saturated fats are solid at room temperature, and they're also pretty darn stable. Saturated fats usually are slower to go rancid or become oxidized than unsaturated fats.

As with all foods that come from an animal, the quality of the fat depends on what the animal eats. Organic butter has a deeper color and contains a different blend of nutrients (including anti-inflammatory omega-3 fatty acids) than con- ventional butter because the cows that produce the milk for organic butter eat much more grass than grains. Organic butter also contains much higher levels of conjugated linoleic acid (CLA) and butyric acid, which are both notable fats that may have anticancer potential.

Don't be fooled by the media-driven nonsense about saturated fats. You need some in your diet every day.

Unsaturated Fats

Monounsaturated fats are missing just one hydrogen atom. They're liquid at room temperature but solidify in the fridge. Foods high in monounsaturated fats are olive oil, avocados, and many nuts.

Polyunsaturated fats are missing more than one hydrogen atom, so they're always liquid, even at colder temperatures. They can also spoil a lot faster than other types of fats. The food industry has solved this problem by refining the heck out of corn, soy, and other vegetable oils. Highly processed oils can stay fresh for a long time but are highly inflammatory to your body.

Unsaturated oils can go rancid easily because the unsaturated spots on the fatty acid chains are weak points that can be "attacked" by oxygen. Bitter taste is a sign of rancidity. Storing unsaturated oil in a dark glass bottle at cool temperatures can lengthen its shelf life.

Omega-3 and omega-6 are the most famous polyunsaturated fats because they're essential, and they play vital roles in your immune system.

- Omega-3 fatty acids (O3) are needed for your body to make the anti-inflammatory prostaglandin PGE3. The body uses inflammation for healing, and it needs PGE3 to clean up that inflammation. Without enough omega-3s in your diet, you can have inflammatory issues, like low-grade chronic inflammation.

- Omega-6 fatty acids (O6) have been given a bad name over the last twenty years. They're necessary for making prostaglandin E1 (PGE1) and prostaglandin E2 (PGE2). PGE1 is a forgotten but important anti-inflammatory prostaglandin, and PGE2 is pro-inflammatory and necessary, so the immune system can trigger inflammation for healing.

The key here is balance. You need the right amount of these fats for your immune system to work correctly. But for decades, food manufacturers have been using highly refined, pro-inflammatory omega-6 oils (like corn and soy oils) to replace saturated fat in their foods. This practice makes the Nutrition Facts label on food products fall in line with the warning to stay away from saturated fat, but it's also skewed the average O6-to-O3 ratio. In 1900, people had about two times the O6 in their diets as they had O3. On average, people today consume about twelve times as much O6 as O3! No wonder inflammation is running rampant right now!

Healthy Fats

Adding more healthy fat to your diet can make your skin glow and your hair shine, and it can help every cell in your body work better. Go, healthy fat!

As a rule of thumb, healthy fat is always an unprocessed or just-barely-processed fat. The farther away from its original nature-made form a fat gets, the more problematic it can be. If you think about fats being on a spectrum, the most natural fat is found in food (like the fat in avocados), and the most unhealthy and unnatural fat is the refined and then chemically altered trans fat. Try getting your dietary fat from the following sources:

- **Healthy fatty foods:** Avocado, raw nuts and seeds, olives, wild cold-water fish (if cooked at less than 350°F), dark chocolate (because it's full of cocoa butter), and free-range eggs. Good quality cheese made from grass-fed milk is also a healthy fatty food, but cheese made from modified milk ingredients is not (not all cheese is equal).

- **Healthy oils and butter:** Cold-pressed oils like extra-virgin olive oil, hemp seed oil, and flaxseed oil (but use hemp or flax oil only for cold applications; don't heat them). Virgin coconut oil and organic butter are beautiful saturated fats. Avocado oil and grapeseed oil are probably okay to cook with (but experts disagree about this).

Stay far away from highly processed and refined oils like vegetable oil, canola oil, refined palm oil, refined sunflower and safflower oils (although cold-pressed sunflower or safflower oil is okay), and all types of margarine.

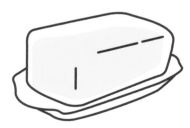

PROTEIN: TODAY'S BIGGEST FAD

Protein is the building block of life. It's often thought of as a muscle builder, but it does so much more than that. Protein is also a major component of bones, teeth, hair, and nails. (Yes, bones consume a lot of dietary protein!) As important as protein is, the hype about it is a bit much. Here's some protein reality:

Protein is a collection of twenty-two amino acids, and your body uses these amino acids to make your muscles and bones. Your body also uses amino acids to create other molecules like hormones, enzymes, neurotransmitters, and antibodies. Protein is a critical factor for growth and repairing the daily wear and tear of your body.

Nine amino acids are considered essential, which means your body can't make these particular amino acids. Another four are conditionally essential because your body can manufacture them sometimes but not at others (like in childhood). The other amino acids are nonessential because your amazing body can create them as long as you're getting enough of the necessary nutrients.

Right now, many nutrition conversations focus on telling people to get more protein. Yes, some people could benefit from more protein, but most people in the Westernized world aren't protein deficient. If anything, many people eat too much protein. Most protein deficiencies are due to digestive issues, *not* a lack of food. Protein from food has to be fully digested and assimilated for your body to access it. So, if you have a digestion or assimilation problem, you can't solve a problem of protein deficiency just by eating more protein; despite the extra protein in your diet, you'll still be protein deficient. And if you eat a high-protein diet while you have issues with protein digestion or assimilation, you may develop more digestive problems and maybe even some food sensitivities.

Vegans and some vegetarians are among the people in Western societies who need to give special consideration to eating enough protein. If you're in this group, you may be familiar with the concept of "protein combining." The idea is to make sure your body receives all nine essential amino acids each day. All animal-derived protein, like meat, dairy, and eggs are complete, but there aren't many complete proteins in a vegan

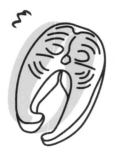

diet. Beans contain some of the essential amino acids, and grains, nuts, and seeds provide the other ones. Very simply, you need to eat one complete protein each day or have beans plus grains, nuts, and/or seeds each day. When you consume all the essential amino acids in a day, then your body can use the amino acids in the rest of your diet. It's an all or nothing situation; you're unable to use any of the protein you've eaten in a day if you don't consume all of the essential amino acids. Pretty much every food—even fruit—has at least some protein. Proper protein combining is an important concept for anyone following a plant-based diet because the need for beans can be easily forgotten.

How Much Protein Do You Need?

The ratio of how many grams of protein a person needs based on body weight has changed many times during my twenty years in the nutrition world. It's gone up and down, and sometimes it's gone *way* up. I like to take a more conservative approach. I find that eating a moderate amount of protein is kinder to the body, and the moderate quantity means you can stay consistent no matter what the current trends suggest you do.

Right now, the Recommended Dietary Allowance (RDA) to prevent protein deficiency is 0.36 gram for every pound of body weight (0.8 gram for each kilogram). However, this quantity of protein is just to *avoid* a deficiency; it's not necessarily the ideal amount.

I usually recommend closer to 0.5 gram for each pound, which means a 150-pound person should aim to eat 75 grams of protein per day (a little at a time rather than all in one meal, which would stress out the digestive system).

What would 75 grams of protein look like? It depends, and that's one of the problems with counting and using numbers: It's hard to translate a number like 75 grams into real-life terms. Most of the time, you don't need to worry about counting anything. Your body will guide you to the right balance.

To hit 75 grams of protein per day, aim for just over 20 grams of protein in each meal and 15 grams in a snack. Some examples of foods that amount to 20 grams of protein are three large eggs, 3 ounces of chicken, 1¼ cups of black beans, or 1½ cups of full-fat yogurt. Plant-based protein sources are less protein-dense, making it a bit trickier to get to 75 grams of protein, but it's still possible.

If you're concerned that your protein intake might be too low, you can track it for a few days to see how much you're eating. My favorite (free) tracking tool is MyFitnessPal. Both the app and the website are easy to use and have many healthy foods already in the database. You can use this tracker, or one like it, for only a few days to see where you are with your protein intake. However, tracking food every day will take you away from paying attention to your body's signals and put your rational mind in charge, so I don't recommend that you do it for an extended time. As I explain in Part 3, your rational mind doesn't quite know what it's doing when it comes to food.

If you're not sure whether you're eating too little or too much protein, look to your body to find out. There are a few particular signs and symptoms that can help you judge your protein intake.

Protein Deficiency

Since you can't take a journey inside your body to check out how your cells, muscles, and bones are doing, you need to use more visible body parts to see how your body is assimilating protein.

Hair and nails need a lot of protein to look healthy, but those features aren't necessary for life. Consequently, you'll detect even a minor protein deficiency in your hair and nails because your body prioritizes other more important body mechanisms, like keeping you strong and making enzymes, over making a glorious mane of hair or beautifully strong nails.

Protein is a building block for many immune system molecules, like antibodies, and sometimes a weaker immune system can be a result of a protein deficiency. You might find that you're getting sick more often or that you feel weaker or more fatigued than usual. For some people, feeling hungry right after eating a meal may be a sign of eating too little protein. Adults over seventy especially need to pay attention to their protein intake because of a natural weakening of the digestive system.

The first and most important stage of protein digestion/assimilation happens in your stomach. The acid in your stomach breaks down protein, and you need a lot of acid to break down protein properly. Stress can weaken the stomach over time, and the production of acid declines. Medications, especially the ones used to treat acid reflux, dilute stomach acid even more. The medicine may stop the burning of your esophagus (which is significant), but it also makes it harder for your body to break down protein because it lowers the amount of acid in the stomach to the point that the acid can't do its job.

Symptoms of low stomach acid include a feeling of heaviness near your ribcage after you've eaten, staying full for a long time after eating, symptoms of protein deficiency, and symptoms of iron and calcium deficiencies. (Both iron and calcium require lots of acid for assimilation.)

In Chapter 9, when I dive deeper into the ins and outs of the digestive system, I outline a few easy steps you can follow to help your protein digestion.

Protein Overconsumption

I commonly hear, "I think I eat too many carbs," but I don't think I've ever heard anyone say, "I think I eat too much protein." Protein has been given such a golden halo of perfection, that it can feel like you can't get enough, but overconsuming protein can be a problem.

An early sign that you're eating more protein than your digestive system can handle is a heavy feeling in your stomach after meals and having gas that smells like sulfur (or rotten eggs). All protein molecules contain some sulfur, and that sulfur-smelling gas is the result of undigested protein in your intestines.

If your body can't digest and assimilate all of the protein you consume, then your body stores the extra as fat. Yes, protein can cause weight gain (gasp)! Researchers have found that protein is more apt to cause weight gain when people replace carbohydrates with protein. So, current food fashions that promote a low-carb, high-protein diet have a few holes in the logic.

High-protein/low-carb diets also are associated with chronic bad breath, constipation, and dehydration. Protein has a diuretic effect and triggers your body to release a bunch of water, which is where a lot of your initial weight loss comes from when you start one of these diets. Remember, if you've suddenly lost a few pounds overnight, I'm sorry to say that those weren't real pounds of fat; you just lost some extra water, which will come back as soon as you increase your carb intake. Any time you observe a fast weight loss or weight gain, it's probably just a shift in water in your body.

Wrapping It All Up

If there's one thing to take from this chapter it's this: Carbs, fat, and protein are all very important. The idea that one is "bad" or another is "good" is just plain ridiculous and sinister.

It's sinister because food fads are used to manipulate your mind so you'll ignore your body's signals and buy into whatever food or diet is popular right now. There's a lot of money to be made in the food product industry when the manufacturers can remove something from a food (first fat, now carbs) and when they can add another thing (now protein, soon to be fat). When you can recognize the wonders of each of these macronutrients and realize that your body needs some of each every day, then you can walk away from food fads for good and embrace the way of eating your body wants.

Now you know that all macronutrients are vitally important for your body to be happy, so you might be wondering how we got to this place where one nutrient or another always seems to be considered "bad." How did eating a healthy diet move from simply eating and enjoying whole food to a complex system of adding up abstract nutrients? In the next chapter, I explain how politicians used flawed logic and flawed nutritional research to create the last four decades of (very misguided) nutritional guidelines.

chapter 6

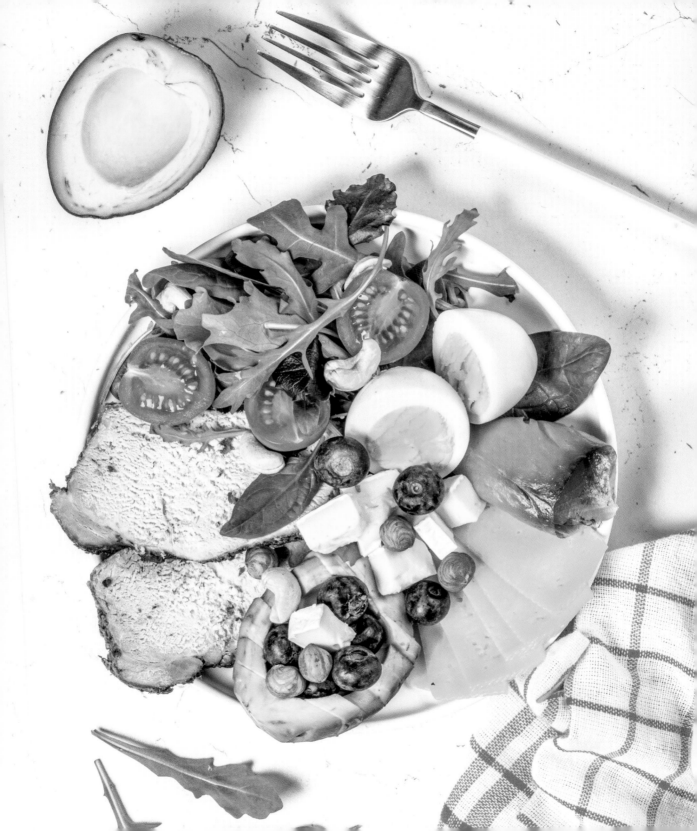

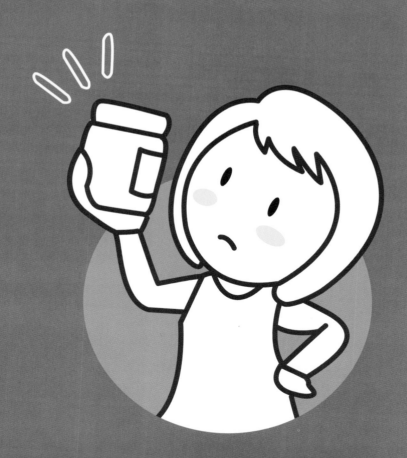

BEWARE FOODS LABELED *HEALTHY*

When people discuss healthy eating, why do they rarely talk about actual food? The conversation tends to center around the parts of food, like, "I'm on a low-carb diet," or, "How do I get more calcium?" Rarely does anyone talk about real food like leafy greens, sweet potatoes, and rice.

The ideology of changing this conversation is *nutritionism,* which is a term coined by professor Gyorgy Scrinis from the University of Melbourne. In a fairly short amount of time (just a few decades), the conversation about diet has turned from something tangible and easy to understand, namely whole foods, to abstract concepts, like nutrients and chemical components. With this change in language, the group of people considered to be food experts has also shifted. Instead of paying attention to their bodies and following inner guidance from hunger cues and taste preferences, most people rely on food manufacturers, national food guides, politicians, nutritionists, dietitians, and researchers.

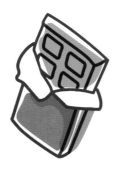

Through this seemingly small change in the way people relate to the food they eat, they've quickly negated their inner wisdom. You may have heard that you should eat every two to three hours, even if you're not hungry. You may have been told to follow a specific style of eating, like low-fat or high-protein, regardless of how you feel when you eat this way. To make things worse, the experts that people rely on to explain what's best keep changing their minds. Instead of paying attention to your innate sense of how to eat, you probably feel bewildered and confused.

Talking about the components of food instead of whole food also makes it possible to plop nutrients into "good" and "bad" categories. For every good nutrient, there must be a villain, right? *Eat less fat and more carbs*, or *eat fewer carbs and more protein*. As a result, food—a real thing you interact with many times a day—has turned into a math equation. Who wants to weigh and measure their food all day long just to make sure they're eating a balanced and healthy diet? I sure don't!

In the not-so-distant past, humans mostly ate whole foods because that was what was available. Food wasn't considered healthy or unhealthy; it was just food. Now, though, nutritionism requires that you understand the abstract concepts of food, such as whether beans are proteins or starches. Do avocados belong in the fatty food category or fiber category?

The truth is that all food has many parts, including parts no one has discovered yet, and reducing any food down to one thing is impossible. Beans are both a source of protein and a healthy starchy food. Avocados are full of healthy fat, *and* they have the most fiber of any fruit. Whole foods don't fit neatly into black-and-white categories, and trying to pigeon-hole them just makes eating confusing.

The big question is, how did we get here in the first place? What happened to shift us so far away from trusting ourselves when it comes to making food decisions? In this chapter, I share how profits and political motivations have convinced people to choose engineered food products over whole-food options for generations.

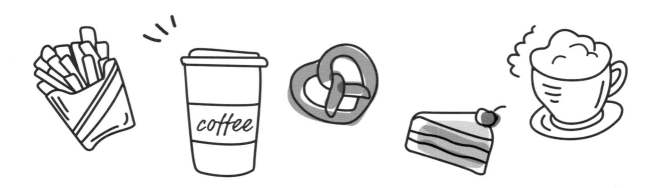

How Did We Get Here?

How did we become so reductionist when it comes to food? Well, it all began with William Prout, the first nutritional scientist.

In the early 1800s, Prout, who was a doctor and chemist, discovered the three macronutrients: carbohydrates, fat, and protein. German scientist Justus von Liebig added a few minerals to the mix, and then he declared he'd found the secret to food. Oh, if only that were true! Liebig used the information to create the first baby formula, but doctors quickly realized that babies who received this formula exclusively didn't thrive. The formula was missing many vitamins, some significant amino acids, and some essential fats that babies need for proper development. The deficient formula was a meaningful sign that there was more to be discovered about human nutrition.

In 1912, Casimir Funk discovered vitamins, which led to finding the cures for vitamin-deficiency conditions like scurvy and beriberi. Vitamins became mega glamorous, and people began to scarf them down by the handful in the hope that vitamins were the key to the fountain of youth. But many other parts of food, such as essential fats, antioxidants, and phytonutrients, were still mysteries at that time, so the picture wasn't complete.

We've come a long way since 1912, but the truth is that nutritional science is a relatively new field, and researchers are still discovering elements of food. With each discovery, it seems like maybe the secret to food has been uncovered. Spoiler—it hasn't.

You only have to look at the times the story has flip-flopped from one nutrient superhero or villain to another to know that the theories have been wrong many times. We now know that it was wrong to vilify fat in the 1980s, and I believe we'll begin to see many repercussions of the low-carb diet very soon. Carbs aren't the superhero experts thought they were in the '80s, and I expect we'll begin to see the dark side of high-protein diets soon enough. What I find the most frustrating about the flip-flopping of nutritional science is that it has stolen our ability to pay attention to our inner knowledge of what is healthy for us.

Food Manufacturers, Politics, and Money

Food manufacturers think the nutritionism movement is great. They love that they can manufacture foods that fit perfectly within the parameters of any currently popular diet and profit off of the latest "healthy lifestyle" scheme.

For example, in the 1980s, manufacturers removed fat from their foods and started to advertise how healthy their products were—low-fat, low-cholesterol, high-fiber, etc. The implied promises on the labels encouraged people to ignore their natural body cues and buy these "healthy" manufactured foods. Shoppers exchanged rich-tasting whole milk for low-fat skim milk (or the even more processed skim milk powder).

Unfortunately, low-fat foods tend to taste a bit like cardboard, so the manufacturers sweetened them with sugar to enhance the flavor.

There are always repercussions when humans manipulate a food to make it "better." In the example of low-fat dairy products, more recent research has found that the fat in milk is important for blood sugar regulation and is a key player in the absorption of calcium and vitamin D. Oops.

For manufacturers to be able to call out the health benefits of a food, it must come in a package or have a label, and it usually needs an advertising budget—all of which costs money. So, you can assume that the food manufacturers need to cut costs or increase the price. Unfortunately, it's hard for consumers to spot how manufacturers have manipulated the food because the product labels always scream out a health benefit. For example, the packaging for a processed cereal made from cheap refined grain boasts that it's full of added fiber, or a label on yogurt made from highly processed skim milk, a by-product of cream production, may brag that it's low in fat.

Whole foods, like fruits and veggies, typically don't have any packaging to advertise their health prowess. They lack labels that tell you about their high fiber content or their mega antioxidants. Even whole foods packaged in bags and boxes, such as beans and whole grains, rarely boast about their health benefits, and it's unusual that you see a print ad or TV commercial about them.

The effort food manufacturers have put into labeling products with "health-promoting" promises designed to ensnare the average consumer has made it almost impossible for people to be able to shop for groceries unless they have a degree in nutritional science. Grocery shopping is a stressful and confusing journey because food manufacturers have made it so.

Flawed Nutritional Studies

I've joked many times that I can find a nutritional study to support any concept, diet, or health idea I want. Although this statement is a bit tongue in cheek, it's also true (unfortunately). Every wild new diet usually has a study or two that "proves" it.

Many nutrition studies are observational and identify connections along the lines of, "If someone eats less meat, do they have less heart disease?" Observational studies suffer from a bunch of core issues, such as the healthy eater bias, correlations that don't prove causation, and inaccuracy of food frequency questionnaires.

I'll first talk about the healthy eater bias. Observational studies typically look for a correlation between one thing and another (like meat-eating and heart disease). However, your whole diet affects your health, and it's not just one item that upsets the balance. For example, take someone who eats small portions of meat alongside lots of vegetables and whole grains and who exercises regularly. In an observational study, this person's lower meat intake would be incorrectly "observed" as being responsible for their lower risk of heart disease, whereas the 360-degree view of their total health practices would show that the other factors also play a part.

Another significant issue with observational studies is that correlation doesn't mean causation. In other words, just because someone eats more meat and has a higher chance for heart disease doesn't mean the meat is the factor that increased their risk. A meat-eater could have several dietary issues or lifestyle habits that caused heart disease; that person might drink a lot of soda or eat a lot of fast food, or they might have a very stressful job. Humans' diets and lifestyles are too complex to place the blame for problems on one single thing.

Harvard University student Tyler Vigen has put together a hilarious website called Spurious Correlations (tylervigen.com/spurious-correlations) as a reminder that correlation doesn't prove causation. He has found some amazing correlations in observational studies. For example, people who consume margarine are more likely to get divorced, and the U.S. per capita cheese consumption correlates with the number of people who've died by getting tangled in their bedsheets each year. It probably seems obvious that margarine doesn't cause divorce, and cheese doesn't increase the chance of getting tangled in the bedsheets, so remember that diet-based observational studies also tend to confuse correlation with causation.

A third issue with most studies is that researchers use food frequency questionnaires to collect data. Participants fill out a questionnaire monthly (or sometimes just yearly) to tell the researchers about their diets. If you try listing all the food you ate last week, you'll begin to see how unreliable the accuracy of these questionnaires can be.

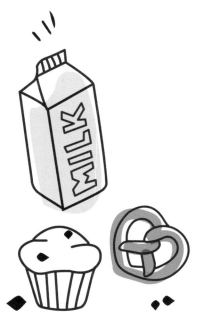

The only way to determine accurate correlation between nutrition and health outcomes would be to lock a group of people inside a metabolic ward where all of their food is measured, and the participants' activities are documented for ten to twenty years. And that's not gonna happen anytime soon.

Because of the inherent flaws in most nutritional studies, I've become very picky with the research I look at for reliable information. I like to look at traditional diets and large population or cohort studies to find some truth.

One example of research that I believe has some validity is a meta-analysis (an analysis of many studies) from 2010 that looked at data from almost 350,000 people. This analysis found no correlation between saturated fat and heart disease, disproving a connection experts had been considering as fact for at least three decades. Meta-analyses suffer from a few controversies, particularly that researchers may pick studies that fit their personal biases and hypotheses, but I like this one because of the sheer number of participants.

Overall, I look at traditional diets as the source for the best information. The diets that have kept human beings healthy for generations provide the best long-term information we have. These diets focus on whole foods (since processed food is a relatively new development) and are balanced for the climate and the season of the location where a person lives. Traditional diets vary from area to area, but overall, they're beautifully balanced whole-food diets. It's just that simple.

The Focus on Single Nutrients

If nutritional science is flawed, and whole-food diets are healthiest, then why does conventional wisdom say to eat more of one nutrient and less of another?

The short answer is *politics*. In the 1970s, nutritionists and the government were concerned about the population's increasing rates of heart disease and felt that something needed to change. The American Heart Association (AHA) had been recommending that people reduce meat and dairy consumption for a few decades. AHA based its recommendations on the lipid hypothesis, which is the idea that fat is bad for health. Dr. Ancel Keys created the lipid hypothesis, and although he didn't prove it conclusively at the time he developed the theory, the lipid hypothesis was considered to be nutritional fact. (The theory has since been disproved.) To decide if the recommendations based on the lipid hypothesis were right for the American public, the U.S. Senate put together a committee to look at the connection between diet and diseases like cancer, heart disease, and obesity. Senator George McGovern was the chairperson.

After two days of listening to testimony, the committee staff (made up of lawyers and journalists rather than doctors or scientists) concluded that the rising meat consumption was to blame for worsening health. In 1977, the committee drafted its first dietary guidelines and told Americans to cut down on dairy and meat.

However, the dairy and beef industries didn't like this conclusion one bit and coerced the committee to change the wording of the recommendations. Instead of the straightforward food recommendation to eat less meat and dairy, the new guidelines pointed to an invisible nutrient: saturated fat. Even "eat less" was removed from the statement and replaced with "choose meats, poultry, and fish that will reduce saturated fat intake."

This development created a massive shift in how people talk about food, and it all came about to keep the food lobbyists and industry happy. From this moment forward, the conversation about food became focused on good or bad nutrients rather than on the food itself. And the recommendations rarely say to eat less of a particular food; they say to eat more of a nutrient deemed to be beneficial (like unsaturated fat). Even refined white sugar wasn't put into the "eat less" category until very recently, and the sugar lobby is still fighting that categorization.

When the committee members made that little change in language in the recommendations, they also made it harder to eat whole food. Let's say you're aiming to hit the 25 to 30 grams of daily fiber that the government recommends. You'd have a hard time measuring your fiber intake while eating a whole-food diet because fiber is invisible, and it's impossible to know the fiber content of every food you eat. The handy Nutrition Fact label on packaged foods was designed to make determining those numbers easier. Unfortunately, food manufacturers can manipulate those nutrition facts.

Unfortunately for Senator McGovern, changing the language of the dietary recommendations didn't save his political career. In the next election, the beef lobby succeeded in removing this three-term senator, which sent a clear message to every politician: *Don't mess with the food lobbies.*

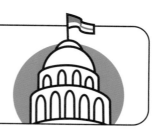

The Misleading Nutrition Facts Label

I can't count the number of times someone has asked me to put together a presentation to teach a group how to read the Nutrition Facts label. This confusing little box is an Achilles' heel for so many people who are trying to be healthier. The Nutrition Facts label tells you all about those invisible components of food that you've been told to pay attention to, but it won't tell you how healthy a food is.

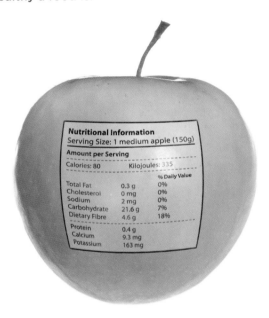

Nutritional Information
Serving Size: 1 medium apple (150g)

Amount per Serving

Calories: 80	Kilojoules: 335

		% Daily Value
Total Fat	0.3 g	0%
Cholesterol	0 mg	0%
Sodium	2 mg	0%
Carbohydrate	21.6 g	7%
Dietary Fibre	4.6 g	18%
Protein	0.4 g	
Calcium	9.3 mg	
Potassium	163 mg	

To make the contents of a label more attractive, food manufacturers might manipulate the ingredients. For example, to lower the naturally occurring saturated fat in yogurt, manufacturers process the yogurt to reduce the fat, which changes the taste, so they increase the sugar and add some thickeners to make it taste better. In the end, the saturated fat is lower, but is the product with added sugar and thickeners healthier than the original that had more fat?

When you want to determine how healthy a food is, you'd do better to look at the list of ingredients on a food package than the Nutrition Facts label. The ingredients list quickly gives you a good indication of how processed the item is. There's a huge difference between a box of muesli and a snack cake. Or a can of beans and a loaf of white bread.

When you look at the ingredients list, ask yourself if you recognize each ingredient as a food. Do you see chemical names scattered throughout? Chemical names are usually a sign of a highly processed food. Some exceptions are tocopherols (vitamin E) and ascorbic acid (vitamin C) that are used as natural preservatives.

The ingredients are listed in order from the most to the least. The top three ingredients usually make up most of that food, so take a good look at those. Food manufacturers can be a little tricky about added sugar. They don't want to list any type of sugar in the top three because they know people are on the lookout for sugar. Instead, manufacturers use multiple types of sugar—like maple syrup, cane sugar, and brown rice syrup—so each ingredient can be listed separately and give the buyer the impression that sugar isn't as significant as it is. All of these ingredients are okay types of sugar, but when used in combination, the quantity can be a *lot* of added sugar! So, watch out for this trick.

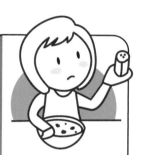

Some labeling laws allow for the trans fat to be rounded down to 0 gram, so a product may include some added trans fat even though the Nutrition Fact label states 0 gram.

There *is* a time to look at the Nutrition Facts label. If you see varieties of sugar listed more than once in the ingredients list, check out the sugar entry on the label to see how many grams of sugar are included. (I hope "added sugar" will get its own listing someday.) Also, take a look at trans fat and avoid any food that includes trans fat or hydrogenated oils in the ingredients. Also, check out the panel if you've been told by your doctor to keep an eye on your sodium or potassium consumption, the Nutrition Facts label can help you watch out for that.

Remember, as a general rule, focus on the ingredients rather than the Nutrition Facts label. Most important, remember that the best foods (like apples) don't have an ingredients list or a Nutrition Facts label.

Wrapping It All Up

Food politics and nutritionism have steered people away from listening to the inner voice that tells them what their bodies want to eat.

I think the most important thing that nutritionism has stolen is pure food pleasure and joy. When you're too busy thinking about what you should and shouldn't eat, you ignore what it is that you *want* to eat and what feels right to eat. Even worse, worrying about nutritionism can make you feel guilty about eating the foods you enjoy.

The good news is that you can choose to leave nutritionism at any time and start looking at food as a whole again. Whole-food eating is an easy way to achieve a healthy diet that's filled with pleasure and joy.

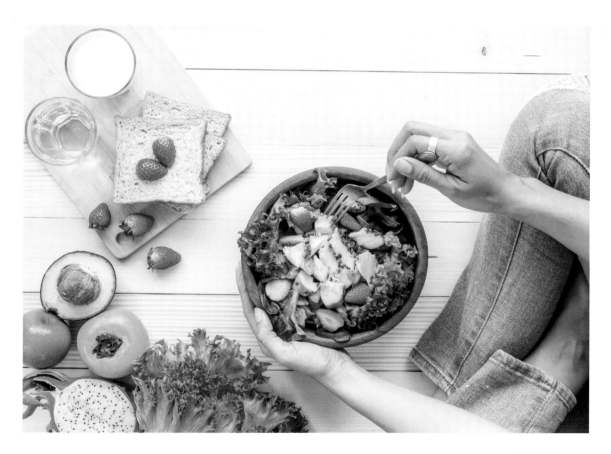

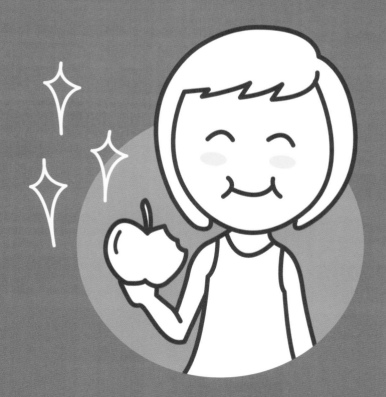

THE SIMPLICITY OF WHOLE FOODS

In this age of confusion and frustration and with the concept of nutritionism making things so complex, could healthy eating actually be simple?

The short answer is yes. Yes, it can.

If you look back at the traditional diets that kept your ancestors healthy for multiple generations, you can find some answers. First, they ate whole foods. Second, they ate the food that was available to them; in other words, they ate according to the seasons and the climate where they lived.

I know; those "rules" of eating seem way too simplistic. What about all the things researchers have uncovered about food? If you follow only those two simple guidelines, how do you make sure your diet is healthy? And balanced in minerals? And has enough protein?

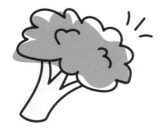

Those concerns are fair, but consider this: Humans were arguably much healthier when it comes to preventable diet-related diseases, like cardiovascular disease and diabetes, before knowing anything about protein and nutrients. Before anyone had identified what a calorie was, obesity was rare. It seems that once people started counting calories and paying attention to these abstract and invisible components of food, the health of the general population went downhill.

There's no question that life expectancy is higher today than it was 100 hundred years ago. In 1900, the average person born in the U.S. lived for only about 47 years because infectious diseases like pneumonia, flu, and tuberculosis were the top three major causes of death. In the last century, medical advances, like antibiotics, have increased the life expectancy in the United States to more than 78 years old. Now, the problem is newer "modern" conditions that are cutting years off our lives. Chronic diseases such as cardiovascular disease and diabetes—many of which have a lifestyle or diet connection to health—are common causes of death.

I believe there's only one simple nutritional idea to focus on, and that's nutrient density. If you focus on eating nutrient-dense foods, you'll automatically shift your diet to unprocessed whole foods. And because your body inherently understands whole foods, it can guide you to the balance of food that your beautiful and unique body needs.

Eating a nutrient-dense whole-food diet is a straightforward answer, but it's not a quick fix. It's a long-term solution for a long-term problem; this approach is how you keep your body healthy for decades. You won't drop any excess weight quickly, but the weight loss is much more likely to be permanent. This concept isn't a diet or a cleanse. It's a way to live every day. By shifting your diet toward whole foods and by learning your body's language of eating, you'll move off the dieting treadmill and into real-life healthy eating.

Plus, a significant side effect (and benefit) of eating a nutrient-dense whole-food diet is food *freedom*. No more dieting, counting, obsessing, and confusion because you'll understand your body so well that you'll know exactly what to eat. Joy and pleasure replace those old frustrations. Food freedom is seriously good eats.

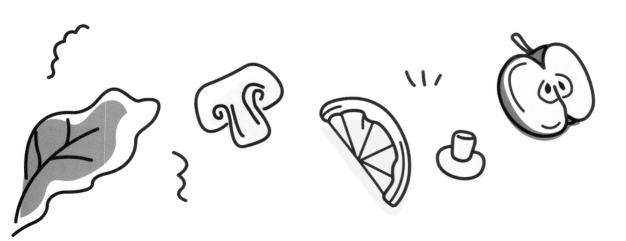

What Are Whole Foods?

Humans have been cooking and preparing food for about 200,000 years, but refining food, or isolating parts of a whole food, is relatively new. Chemically refined sugar was first processed in India about 2,500 years ago, but until the last 100 years or so, refined sugar and flour were considered rare and expensive rather than an everyday ingredient. Cakes and sweet treats made from white flour and white sugar were a delicacy available only to the upper classes until the late 1800s. Before that time, people had to satisfy a sweet tooth with in-season fruit or a lucky opportunity to steal some honey away from the bees.

Just a few generations ago, all food was relatively whole. What would your great-great-grandparents think about your current eating habits? I don't think they'd be very impressed. Although I'm grateful that I don't have to spend all day preparing the family meal, I believe that a lot of people have lost the pleasure and enjoyment that comes from eating a well-earned meal. Fast food and fast eating have turned something that used to be a pleasurable gathering into a job to get done as quickly as possible.

Whole foods are foods that look the same as they did when they came out of the ground or from an animal—fruits, vegetables, whole grains, nuts, seeds, beans, eggs, meats. Traditionally processed foods, such as fermented foods, canned vegetables, milk, whole milk yogurt, cheese, cold-pressed oils, and traditionally rendered fat (like butter) are also whole foods. I like to lump frozen fruits and veggies into the category. Even though freezing isn't a traditional process, it involves minimal processing, and frozen food retains more of its nutrients than canned food.

You can use someone who lived in the 1800s as a guide to what a whole food is because it's a food they would recognize. Any food processing they would have done, like canning, fermenting, or milling, can usually be considered a healthy process. Foods that have been through those processes usually still look very much like they did when they were freshly harvested. Imagine what one of your ancestors would think about a bowl of nacho-flavored tortilla chips—an unnaturally orange food that bursts with lab-made flavor and contains many chemical additives. I don't think they'd guess those chips were food at all.

Another way to know if a food is whole is by looking at its shelf life. Does it rot? Does it spoil quickly? If the answer is yes, then it's probably a whole food. The refining of food, like flour, sugar, and oils, have given many processed foods an unbelievably long shelf life. White flour and white sugar can be five, ten, or even fifteen years old and still look and smell like they're fresh. (But please don't eat food that old, even if it looks okay.) Whole wheat flour, on the other hand, spoils so quickly that I've rarely been able to find it at my grocery store before it's gone rancid.

The food processors benefit financially from these foods with a long shelf life, but those foods don't provide any benefit to the consumers.

I have one extra category I like to include under the whole-food umbrella: "minimally processed" foods, which are packaged or convenience foods made from real food. Hummus and muesli are examples. You could make these foods at home, but it's nice to let someone else make them for you sometimes. In this category, all of the items in the ingredients list should be recognizable as food.

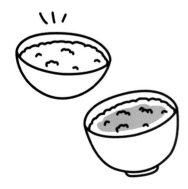

I have one exception to the whole-food rule: Sometimes white rice is better than brown rice. Brown rice as a whole is much more nutrient dense than white rice, but if you look at the nutrients you absorb when you eat rice, white rice is the superior food. The fiber in brown rice is high in phytic acid, a natural antinutrient that can block the absorption of all of the beautiful nutrients in brown rice. Also, fiber is scratchy and hard on sensitive guts, so I usually recommend white rice to anyone who has irritable bowel or other digestive issues. But—and this is important—because white rice is missing its fiber, you should eat it the way people eat it in countries that traditionally eat rice. It should be an accompaniment, *not* the focal point of a meal. In North America, people tend to cover the plate with rice and then put a few veggies in the middle of the rice pile. Instead, flip those measurements. Fill your plate or bowl with veggies and then add a small handful of rice as a healthy starch. When eating brown rice, be sure to soak it overnight (or at least for a few hours) to get rid of the nutrient-blocking phytic acid.

When you eat whole foods, you also avoid myriad chemical additives in processed food. Artificial dyes that are added to everything from breakfast cereals to sports drinks have been linked to behavior issues in children, many preservatives have been linked to cancer, and a variety of food additives disturb the gut bacteria and inflame the gut. Whole foods may not stay fresh for three years, but your body will be happier without these unnecessary chemicals.

What Is Seasonal Eating?

When I was a kid, I waited all year for strawberries to be in season. My grandmother had them in her garden, and I can remember that burst of sweetness when I would dive into a big bowl of her homegrown strawberries or a piece of strawberry shortcake. I'd eat strawberries on almost anything. But then, in a blink of an eye, strawberry season would be over, and I'd have to wait until the next year. (Luckily, peach season was just around the corner.)

Now is an excellent time to be a foodie. Many people live near supermarkets that stock every kind of food imaginable all year long. Kids today don't have to wait for their favorite fruit to be in season; strawberries are available in stores every day. So are salad greens, peas, stone fruits, and all of the foods that used to be hard to store through the winter.

In all this food abundance, it's easy to forget that your body is connected to the seasons. The watery foods that grow in the height of summer, like lettuce, cucumbers, tomatoes, and watermelons, cool you down. And the hardier veggies that are easy to store—potatoes, carrots, and sweet potatoes—are full of slow-burning energy to keep you warm in winter.

Think about how you feel when you eat a big salad in the winter? For one, you probably get cold. Then, if you're like many people, you may find that you have a craving for sugar as your body tries to warm you up.

EATING (AND DRESSING) FOR THE WEATHER

A few years ago, during an unseasonably warm day in February, I was doing an event at a health-food store. The temperature wasn't hot (I live in Canada, after all), but it was well above freezing, and many people were sporting only spring coats. A woman came up to me and wanted to know what I thought about the raw food diet, and I told her the truth: It can be lovely in the summertime, but many people find it difficult in the winter if they live in a colder climate. In the winter, the body usually prefers cooked food, like soups and stews. She furrowed her brow and said, "Darn, I eat a raw food diet, and I was hoping you'd convince my husband that he should eat more raw food. He likes soups, too."

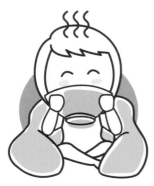

When she walked away, I noticed her outfit. She was in a full parka and snow pants! She was *cold*, possibly because her raw food diet wasn't keeping her warm enough. Later, she approached me again with another question, so I commented on her outfit. She leaned in and said, "You know, you're right. I *am* cold. I wear snow pants in the house."

By shifting what you eat in the fall to warmer foods, you'll find that cold weather is much more tolerable, and you'll probably feel much more satisfied after your meals. It's okay to switch from salads to warm soups in January; it's what your body is asking for.

Seasonal eating assumes that food is more than just a sum of its nutrient parts and that it contributes to your body temperature regulation by being warming or cooling. Before passing this idea off as a far-out, new-agey concept, keep in mind that only Westernized medicine doesn't consider this aspect of food. The idea that food is seasonal and has a warming or cooling nature is found in traditional Chinese medicine and Ayurvedic medicine, and both traditions are more than 5,000 years old.

Until very recently, human beings ate food that was in season and climate-appropriate for their home location; it wasn't possible to ship blueberries from South America or grow hydroponic tomatoes in February. In colder climates, people would have enjoyed root vegetables, hardy fruit like apples and pears, and maybe some fatty meats to stay warm during the winter, and their diets would naturally have lightened up with sprouts and leafy greens in the spring. Summer provided a bounty of ripe berries, fruits, and heat-lovin' veggies like tomatoes and zucchini. The fall harvest offered the harder-skinned veggies, like squash and carrots, that would feed people all winter long.

Many people consider a summery diet to be the healthiest—lots of salads, raw veggies, lean meats, and berries. It's definitely a delicious way to eat. At least it is until the colder winds start to blow in the fall. Light salads with a high water content are very cooling, and they're perfect for meals in August. But in the late fall and winter, they're too cooling for a chilly day.

Your body is wonderfully brilliant, and when the temperature outside turns colder, it wants to rebalance with something warmer, which is usually something sweet or starchy.

You can say no for a while, but eventually, your body will win. You might give in to some comfort food for dinner one night or a plate of cookies during the holidays. Instead of fighting the temptations, there's an easier answer—seasonal eating, which means you eat food that's good for you when that food is *in season*.

A lot of my clients initially struggle in the fall because that light and summery diet stops feeling good, but they always feel guilty about eating and enjoying heavier foods. They have guilty feelings for not wanting to eat a big salad with dinner every night. So, I remind them that their bodies are asking, as politely as possible, for a diet change, and no guilt is necessary.

You might be thinking, "But shouldn't I eat salads and raw veggies no matter what time of year it is? Aren't those foods the healthiest for me? I'm looking to lose weight, so don't I *need* to eat salads?" The answer is both yes and no. Salads are beautifully healthy for you when they're *in season*. But, in the middle of winter, they can increase your cravings for refined sugar and flour, which offsets the health benefits and may bring down your mood.

If you feel great after having a salad, even in the middle of winter, great! Keep it up! However, if you're forcing yourself to eat salads because you "should" eat them, then consider moving to more wintry food. You don't have to master seasonal eating to feel the benefits; small shifts make a huge difference. For me, the wonderful oranges and grapefruit available in January and February really brighten up those cold and dark months. Since I live in Canada, these citrus fruits are not in season for me, but I enjoy them. I also enjoy lots of in-season vegetables like sweet potatoes and beets, which balances my love of citrus fruits.

Eating in-season food is also a very economical way of eating. You may have access to almost every fruit and veggie imaginable all year round, but you pay for this luxury. Strawberries in January might be four or five times the price they are in June, and even the cost of apples skyrockets in the early summer. These foods have to travel thousands of miles from a much warmer climate to arrive on your plate in the winter. Food is much cheaper and more nutrient-dense when it only needs to travel from the farm down the way rather than from halfway around the world.

By shifting your diet each season, you'll find your cravings lessen, and you'll be much more tolerant of the weather. Eating seasonally appropriate foods will help you feel warmer in the winter (especially with a nice bowl of warm soup with some extra warming ginger) and cooler in the heat of the summer (especially if you're like me and try to survive the heat without air-conditioning).

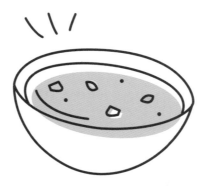

How Do I Shop for Whole Foods?

Switching your diet to a whole-food diet can be easy if you follow the few guidelines I cover in the following sections. As you transition to this way of eating, take your time; don't feel you need to change everything all at once. Moving too quickly will make grocery shopping unnecessarily miserable. If you're starting where I did, with a diet that's mostly processed food, make changes to just one food type at a time. You'll be surprised how easy it'll be and how quickly your cupboards will change!

Shop Around the Edges of the Store

The owners of your supermarket know that produce, bread, meat, eggs, and milk are most likely on your grocery list, but they want you to buy other food. They encourage you to do that by putting the must-have items as far from each other as possible, usually along the edges of the store. Store management would like you to wander up and down the aisles among the processed food as you travel from one side to the other, but you don't have to. Stick to the edges, and you'll be outta there in no time!

Load Up on Veggies and Fruit

The easiest way to change your diet is to focus on adding healthy foods rather than removing unhealthy ones. Extra servings of veggies and fruit will squeeze out any of the foods you'd like to eat less of. Make sure you have all of your favorite healthy foods on your grocery list. If you're new to buying produce, start with fruit that you've enjoyed in the past. Once you've gotten a taste for fresh produce, try some new and easy veggie recipes, like a simple soup, stew, or pan of roasted veggies.

This approach of adding healthy foods instead of subtracting "unhealthy" food does more than just increase your veggie intake. It gives you something positive to focus on because you're *adding* new food to your diet. Dieting culture has trained people to focus on a negative or punitive approach of removing many things from their diets. This undieting method instead helps shift your thinking from negative to positive. This shift may seem small, but it's a significant attitude adjustment that can change the way you look at food forever. Everything is allowable; you just add a bit more of these whole foods. Simplicity for the win!

Replace One Processed Food at a Time with a Healthier Version

Do you love sugary cereal in the morning? Look for a low-sugar granola that you'll love just as much. Do you love sweetened yogurt? Try an unsweetened version and add some honey (or use a half-and-half mix of sweetened and unsweetened yogurt). Do you love ketchup? Look for an option with better ingredients that's sweetened with honey. Does a jar of pasta sauce make for an easy dinner? Look for one without any added sugar or corn starch. Give yourself time for your taste buds to adjust by gradually incorporating healthier versions, and over time you'll start to prefer the new versions to the old.

Ignore the Commercials

The easiest way to tell if a food is a whole food is by whether it has a commercial. As a general rule, whole foods don't receive advertising because the farmers' budgets don't have room for the expense. There are occasional exceptions (the avocado industry has recently been doing some advertising), but whole foods typically don't advertise. In general, only highly processed food is profitable enough to afford an advertising campaign.

Wrapping It All Up

A whole-food diet doesn't have to be a "perfect" diet for it to be healthy. That's what I love about this way of eating.

From the very first whole food you try, your body will always benefit from adding one more. My body cheered when I incorporated my first whole food into my 100 percent processed food diet, and it kept cheering with each new one I added. With each new whole food you try, remember to enjoy every single bite. Whole food loves to be enjoyed.

Don't be surprised if your mind fights back at the simplicity of undieting at first. The dieting culture has spent decades and millions of dollars to put that guilt-ridden little voice inside your head to tell you that you need to follow a strict diet to be healthy. In Part 2, I break down the dieting industry so you can see how profit-driven (not health-driven) its message has always been.

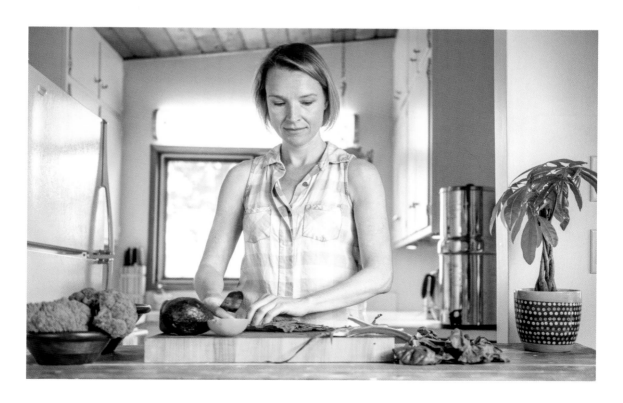

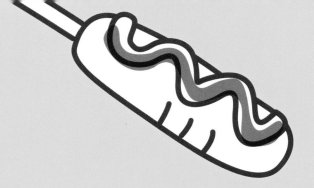

PART **2**

GETTING OUT OF THE DIETING MINDSET

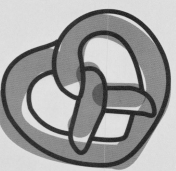

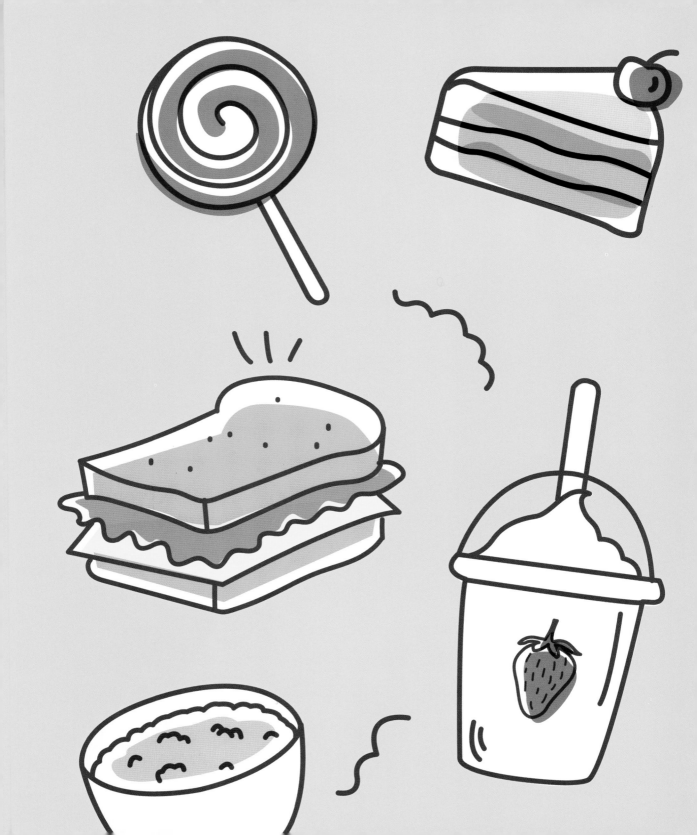

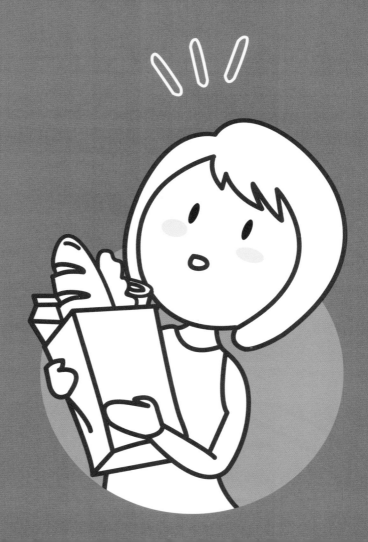

PROFIT-DRIVEN FOOD MANUFACTURING

When you go to a store to buy groceries, you're unintentionally making both health decisions and political decisions. You're voting with each dollar you spend. With your purchases, you can vote for more whole food and ethical growing and agricultural practices, or you can vote for more of the same old, same old.

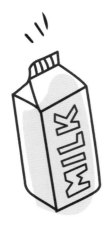

The weight of these decisions can make you feel intimidated when you're in the grocery store. You might be laboring over questions and big choices—which product is healthier? Is the more expensive brand a better option?

The truth is that food manufacturers benefit from your confusion. It enables them to "trick" you into grabbing their product instead of a competitor's. Profits, not your health, are driving the manufacturers' motivations. Consequently, I think it's important that you fully understand the profit-driven decisions food manufacturers and grocery store executives make to arm yourself with the truth so you can see through their trickery.

In this chapter, I break down some of the profit-driven motivations behind many of the products at your grocery store. You'll learn the industry motivations behind federal dietary recommendations and how advertising budgets determine where products are placed on shelves. After reading this chapter, you'll have the tools you need to be able to bypass the tricks to find the best food in the store.

Competition for Your Stomach

Food manufacturers desperately want their products to land in your cart and their food to land in your stomach. The industry term for this is "competing for stomach share." The idea is that a single person can eat only so much in a day, and manufacturers need to compete to have their products be among those foods you choose.

Frankly, farmers of fruits and vegetables also compete for their stomach share, but they don't have the same resources as the food manufacturers. Their produce is usually not subsidized by the government, so their profit margins are lower. They don't have money for big advertising campaigns or even fancy labels.

Food manufacturers, on the other hand, have big (even giant) budgets to advertise their foods. They also have the budgets to pay for firms to lobby government officials to change policies to be favorable to their industry. Lobby groups have encouraged the government to subsidize big staple crops—like corn, wheat, and soybeans—which are the same crops that make up the white flour, high-fructose corn syrup, and vegetable oil that form the base for most processed food. It's no wonder processed food is so darn cheap, whereas fresh vegetables can be so expensive. Big food manufacturers also have helped to shape dietary recommendations, such as the ones that recommend we have more polyunsaturated fat (vegetable oil) and less saturated fat (butter).

I don't believe all food manufacturers are evil companies that are out to do harm everywhere they turn. I'm sure they're run by people who'd love for all of us to be healthier, but the more pressing concern is profit. And there's a lot of profit to be made when companies process and adjust simple whole food to create exciting new food products that conform to whichever food idea is fashionable at the time.

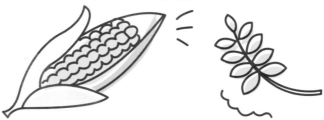

The Food Industry's Profitable Influence on Dietary Recommendations

In the 1980s, food manufacturers did a great job of creating every low-fat food people could dream of! Low-fat milk, yogurt, and cheese replaced whole milk products. Manufacturers added emulsifiers and thickeners in an attempt to simulate the creaminess of whole milk (although it was never quite right). Margarine replaced butter, multi-ingredient Miracle Whip replaced three-ingredient mayonnaise, and many companies even attempted to make low-fat ice cream. What these low-fat foods lacked in flavor, they made up for in added sugar. Because they were fat-free, however, they wore a golden halo of being "guilt-free" or, at least, "better for you." Unfortunately, by the mid-1990s, Americans were heavier than ever. Lower fat did not equal better health or lower weight. Today, although dietary trends acknowledge that good fats are a necessary component of a healthy diet, threads of the low-fat craze are still all over the grocery stores.

In the last few years, new information has come to light about what was happening behind the scenes in the 1960s to inspire the low-fat craze. In the 1950s and 1960s, researchers identified connections between fat intake and heart disease, and they identified a relationship between sugar intake and heart disease. The Sugar Research Foundation (SRF) wanted to shift the conversation away from sugar and push the "fat is bad" agenda. The group hired some Harvard researchers to do a literature review, but the SRF hand-selected the studies that were to be included. Unsurprisingly, the Harvard researchers found problems with all of the studies that vilify sugar and concluded that cutting saturated fat was the best way to reduce Americans' risk of heart disease.

The reviewers did exactly what they were paid to do—shift the conversation away from sugar and place it squarely on fat. In 1967, the literature review was published in *The New England Journal of Medicine*, with no mention of its funding from the sugar industry. This review played a significant role in shaping the dietary recommendations in the 1970s and 1980s and beyond. The authors of the *JAMA* article that exposed this connection in 2016 say that the sugar industry's influence in nutritional research has continued for the last five decades.

Interestingly, getting off the hook for heart disease wasn't the only benefit for the sugar industry. Focusing public attention on reducing fat instead of sugar also brought in a sweet profit. Food devoid of fat becomes bland and unpalatable. Food manufacturers solved this problem by adding extra sugar to make low-fat foods taste better. The SRF president predicted this outcome in 1954 in a speech in which he connected a low-fat diet with higher sugar intake. He estimated that a low-fat diet could increase sugar profits by one-third.

His prediction was right. The sugar consumption of each person in the United States did increase but by much more than one-third. From 1920 to 1954, sugar consumption per capita had declined, but that trend changed in the mid-1950s and made a sharp increase. Between 1955 and 2000, the per capita sugar intake in the United States went up by more than 60 percent!

Problems with the Federal Dietary Guidelines

I firmly believe that the folks in charge of creating the dietary guidelines are trying to do a good job by recommending a healthy diet to follow. The research that they follow may be problematic, but their intent is sound, and they're trying to do some good in the world. Unfortunately, with each new iteration of the guidelines, they've failed.

I believe nutritionism—which focuses on single nutrients rather than the whole food—contributes to the problem. When the dietary experts are limited by having to recommend that the public eat more or less of single nutrients rather than focusing on whole food, the window is wide open for food manufacturers to manipulate the recommendations in a way that favors making new products.

By the end of the 1990s, the evidence that eating a low-fat diet may be more harmful than helpful was becoming apparent, and the low-carb, high-protein Atkins diet craze swept in to fill the void. Quickly, foods that had been considered healthy in the 1980s, like pasta and bread, were shunned. Food manufacturers rapidly addressed this problem by reformulating their recipes. Suddenly high-protein bread and low-carb pasta hit the stores. Even though those products had higher prices, consumers were eager to buy them, and the products flew off the shelves. Entire stores dedicated to selling low-carb processed food opened.

Today, views about healthy eating are going through a recalibration. After two decades of protein being royalty, fat has come in to take its crown. Manufacturers are reformulating products to be "keto-friendly" by making them high in fat.

How to Navigate in the Grocery Store

Where does it leave consumers? Well, you might feel like you need a diploma in nutrition just to be able to set foot in a grocery store and come out with healthy food. That confusion is helpful to food manufacturers because it makes it easier for the companies to sell products. This confusion will persist until consumers stop buying the products. This is what I meant at the beginning of the chapter when I talked about voting with the dollars you spend. Refusing to purchase food manufacturers' products influences what they produce and can really make a difference.

When you're shopping, it's important to know about a tricky technique that merchandisers use to influence every decision you make—*nudging*. Richard Thaler, an economics and behavioral science professor at the University of Chicago's Booth School of Business, first described the nudge theory in 2008. The theory states that 80 percent of a person's behavior is automatic, and that automatic or mindless behavior can be used to change a person's buying habits. In 2017, he even won a Nobel Prize in Economic Sciences for this theory!

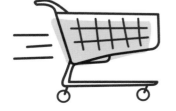

For many years, grocery stores and restaurants have been using these techniques to nudge you toward their more profitable items. Grocery store chains even charge companies for the opportunity to be in a good location. Stores charge a lot more for placement on their eye-level shelves, but only processed food companies can afford this fee. Endcap displays are particularly expensive and are usually filled with highly processed and profitable food. Most healthier food manufacturers just can't compete. One exception is the cereal aisle. The most expensive shelf for product placement is the bottom shelf because it's at a child's eye level. The cereal manufacturers are trying to nudge your child, not you, into wanting their product.

In its simplest terms, nudging, or "choice architecture," means changing an environment to change behavior without making anything forbidden or out of bounds. No one has said you can't eat a certain food; instead, merchandisers put some products (the healthier options) out of reach and place some other products (the highly processed items with the big advertising budgets) closer. That's why the chocolate bars—rather than the apples—stare at you while you pay for your groceries. The chocolate bars have a much better profit margin.

The expense for placement on these eye-level shelves comes directly out of your wallet every time you buy those products. The manufacturing company passes those expenses along to the consumers in two ways: Either the purchase price of the product is a bit higher than a similar quality product, or the product is cheaper to produce than a similarly priced product. (Sometimes, both things are at play.) All food advertising is, at the end of the day, paid for by the consumers. The food executives always make sure their pockets are well lined with your hard-earned cash at the end of the day.

This is why it's so important to vote with your dollar any time you can.

I've got good news for you: Now that you know about the grocery store's little trick, you can find the best quality food on the shelf. Just follow a simple rule: the most profitable food (usually also more expensive and more processed) is at eye level. The less profitable food (usually the *least* processed) is in an inconvenient spot. Look at the top or bottom shelf and at the far ends of each section. I usually find the best muesli or granola on the top shelf and at the very end of the section. The best yogurt is often hiding in the bottom corner at the end of the refrigerated section. Just look a bit out of your way, and you'll find some amazing food!

Wrapping It All Up

Being trained in nutrition helps in the grocery store, but only when you're walking up and down the middle aisles—the ones full of boxes and bags of food. Everything in the produce section is healthy, and you don't need training to buy from that section. Also, you can generally assume that any packaged food that has only a few ingredients, all of which are recognizable, is a relatively healthy food.

When you switch to a whole-food diet, your body will be so much happier, but so will the people in the food industry who produce those foods. Buying a few extra apples this week helps support the farmer who grew them. Grabbing a head of cauliflower or a bag of nuts is a simple way to move away from the political craziness inside the processed food industry. Every whole food you buy is a win.

The grocery store isn't the only place you might find your idea of healthy eating being manipulated. For centuries, one fad diet after another has tried to convince the public that the latest fashionable way of eating will solve every problem. After almost 500 years of dieting, nothing much has changed. Each fad diet is a variation of the last, and all of them exclude essential macronutrients, encourage crash diet routines, or both. The best defense against the next dieting iteration is to understand the full history of fad dieting. By knowing what happened in the past, you can see the future a bit more clearly.

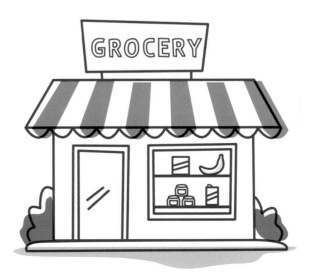

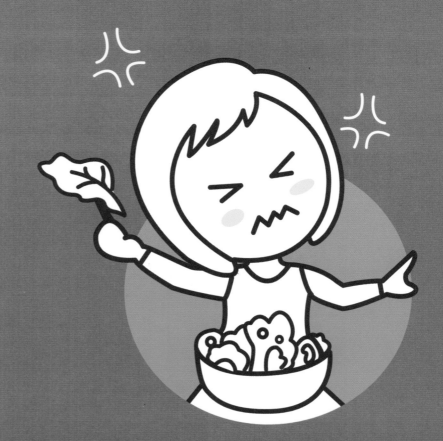

FAD DIETS THROUGH THE AGES

You see a friend that you haven't seen in a while, and the person has totally transformed. They're bright, excited, and noticeably slimmer, and they let you in on their secret. They're following this fantastic new diet that actually works! Does that scenario sound familiar?

Fad diet promoters have encouraged us to try far-out eating techniques for hundreds of years. Whatever new-fangled diet that's out right now, it's just the most recent in a very long line of fad diets. In their time, all fad diets seem at least relatively reasonable and somewhat effective, but not one of these diets has turned into a mainstream way of eating (even though many of them have claimed to be the way everyone would eat in the future).

Between the health experts raving about a diet and friend after friend extolling its virtues, it can be hard not to jump on the bandwagon, too. It's only when you look back in history at the truth of that bright and shiny new way of eating that you see it as a fad diet. Sooner than later, you'll forget about it because another diet will have come to take its place.

In this chapter, I give you a tour through the history of fad dieting, so when the next one rears its ugly head, you can see it for what it is.

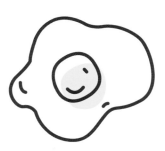

The First Fad Diet

The first recorded diet book that led to a fad diet was published in 1558. Luigi Cornaro wrote *The Art of Living Long* when he was the ripe old age of ninety-one, and he felt that his long life and good health were important topics to write about. In his book, he encouraged "temperance" and eating as little as possible. I believe this is the first low-calorie diet! Although his views were fairly tame and moderate compared to current fad diets, Cornaro was promoting a way of eating that worked for him but wouldn't necessarily work for anyone else.

The poet Lord Byron was the next diet celebrity. His advice was borne out of his vanity. As a famous poet, he was in the public eye, and his obsession with his weight caused him to live on a near-starvation diet. His weight loss and diet were noticed by young socialites, who followed his diet of potatoes, rice, and vinegar to keep their figures. Byron encouraged them by suggesting that "a woman should never be seen eating or drinking, unless it be lobster salad and champagne, the only truly feminine and becoming viands." So, Lord Byron apparently thought a woman was only feminine if she didn't eat. How convenient that he wasn't a woman, so he didn't have to take his own advice.

William Banting, an undertaker, was responsible for the first low-carb diet in the late 1800s. I'm not sure how an undertaker became a dieting expert, but his diet was so popular that his name became a verb; people would commonly say, "I am Banting," to mean, "I'm on a diet." This trend lasted well into the 1920s.

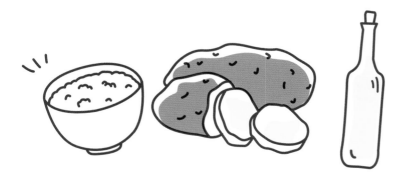

Fad Diets in the 1900s

When I was a kid, our family dinners were a unique affair, although I didn't realize there was anything unusual about them until I spoke with my cousin's wife many years later. When we would eat at my grandparents' farmhouse, we would have a tremendous spread. My grandmother was a fantastic cook, and the table would be covered with a delicious meal, which always included her homemade (and incredibly addictive) rolls. As a family, we'd sit down and dig in.

Once we'd all finished the main course, we'd clear the table and start on dessert. Seems pretty standard, right? It was normal, except for my granddad. Everyone else would have finished eating and moved on to the kitchen to clean up, but my granddad would still be sitting in front of his main dish, chewing away. The head of the household was still eating, all alone at his table.

After my cousin's wife commented about how surprised she was that we would let him finish his meal alone (and I realized that it *was* odd), I asked my dad about his father's very slow eating habits.

My granddad was my first experience with *Fletcherizing,* which was one of the first fad diets of the 1900s. Horace Fletcher, known as "The Great Masticator," promoted a straightforward plan. Eat as much as you'd like, but you must chew each bite 100 times before swallowing. Chewing meticulously is a good practice, although chewing 100 times per bite is overdoing it. (Just chew thoroughly without worrying about counting.) Fletcher's theory of chewing might not count as a fad diet, but it was a practice that went in and out of fashion because most people aren't willing to spend an hour eating every meal. Well, aside from my granddad, who continued to eat his meals slowly for the rest of his life.

The 1920s ushered in the first doctor-promoted diet. In the best-selling book, *Diet & Health: With Key to the Calories,* Dr. Lulu Hunt Peters told women to view every bite of food as calories and not to eat more than 1,200 calories per day. A 1,200-calorie diet, which is almost a starvation diet, is still so popular today that many people see this as a maximum amount to eat in a day instead of what it really is—a bare minimum if you're sitting on the couch all day.

The Cabbage Soup Diet of the 1950s was the advent of the age of the extreme fast-weight-loss fad diets. Today, this type of diet would be called a *cleanse* instead of a *diet* because you're only supposed to follow it for seven days. A week of nothing but cabbage soup, a bit of veggies, and a touch of meat sounds like a very gassy week to me!

The Master Cleanse of the 1990s is a bit of an update of the Cabbage Soup Diet. It's also used for fast weight loss, but it involves a strategy that is like a fast. For ten days, a master cleanser drinks only lemon juice, cayenne, and maple syrup; no food whatsoever is involved. I caution anyone from trying this without first talking to a health practitioner. Some people are great fasters, but for others, fasting can be quite dangerous.

The Dr. Atkins Phenomenon

I came into the health and wellness field in 2002, right at the beginning of the Atkins Diet phenomenon. Although Dr. Robert Atkins published his first book about the diet in 1972 and experienced some success with it, his follow-up book in 2002, *The Diet Revolution*, was what made him a diet celebrity.

This very low-carb, high-protein diet recommended people trade potatoes for bacon, and it included a ketogenic-style intro phase. This diet was hugely popular and even resulted in the opening of many (short-lived) stores that sold Atkins brand low-carb food replacements.

At the time the diet became popular, it was considered a full lifestyle shift, and it was heralded as the diet of the future. I imagine that the popularity of this diet came from its about-face from the low-fat 1980s and 1990s. Eating all the fat you want must have seemed very attractive after people had shunned it for so long. Plus, it was so popular that almost any gathering included one or two people who were scarfing down bacon and losing weight, which made the concept an easy sell. Many other diet books have followed in the footsteps of Atkins, such as the South Beach diet and the Paleo diet, although both diets have promoted eating more veggies than the Atkins diet did.

I believe we can look at the Atkins diet and find some valuable information for evaluating whether any new diet is a fad. The Atkins diet promoted the idea that "you can eat all you want, as long as you shun carbs," which has become a selling point for many current fad diets. Also, the idea was that it could be a lifelong diet and the future way of eating, which are ideas promoted by most fad diets. However, twenty years after the Atkins diet swept the nation, very few people are still following it. I haven't come across anyone following this diet in at least a decade. That's because shunning any macronutrient is nearly impossible for the long term, and, as with every diet, everyone goes back to their normal way of eating eventually. Most people will gain back any weight they lost. It's an unfortunate truth, but it's a truth all the same.

Current Fad Diets

The late 2010s and early 2020s are the age of the ketogenic diet (otherwise known as *keto*). Like the Atkins diet, the keto diet has been massively popular, which has resulted in a movement of supporters who have produced recipe books, food products, and websites.

When followed correctly, the keto diet triggers your body to switch fuel sources. Typically, you burn glucose for energy, which mostly comes from the carbohydrates in your diet. If you dramatically restrict carbs to only about 5 percent of what you eat, then you force your body to use a different source of fuel for energy: ketones.

This ability to switch to burning ketones for fuel is a survival mechanism all humans have, and many keto promoters support the idea that the body runs best on ketones. This belief has yet to be proven, but if by looking at cultures that naturally have times when there aren't any carbs available, we can get an idea whether this is true.

The Inuit live a very low-carb, high-fat lifestyle for many months each year, and researchers have found that the bodies of Inuit people move into ketosis with *much* more difficulty than those people who eat a normal-carb diet throughout their lives. In other words, over time, their bodies have adapted *not* to go into ketosis unless it's absolutely necessary. To me, that doesn't look like ketones are the preferred fuel source, but only time and more research will tell.

The keto diet has been around for decades as a treatment for drug-resistant epilepsy in children. By shifting the body's energy supply from glucose to ketones, this diet can be effective at reducing and sometimes stopping seizures, but this dietary option was always seen as a last resort treatment due to the difficulty in changing the diet to force a person's body to make the switch from burning sugar to burning fat. To stay in ketosis, a person needs to eat a diet that's 70 to 80 percent fat, and getting enough dietary fat to reach 80 percent is both nutritionally difficult to balance and pretty darn unappetizing. I would never have suspected, even ten years ago, that the keto diet would become as popular as it has.

Using keto as a weight-loss method is a pretty new concept that's become wildly popular. Many people swear by it, but many other people experience side effects as nutritional deficiencies, hormonal imbalances, and hair loss. You probably won't be surprised when I say that I'm not a fan of the keto diet.

I have two main arguments against the keto diet:

- It's challenging to balance the diet nutritionally because carbs are where we get most of our vitamins and minerals. So, when you cut out nearly all the carbs, you're inadvertently cutting out a lot of nutritional value.

- It's so hard to stay in ketosis that most people who follow the diet aren't accomplishing that goal. A state of ketosis is a precise math equation: Eat too many grams of carbs or protein, and your body will quickly move back to burning glucose. Pretty much all of the health benefits of the keto diet are from being in the ketogenic state, and I'd argue that many keto dieters are on a nutritionally poor diet without the health benefits of ketosis.

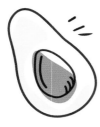

As the ketogenic diet is losing some of its popularity, the carnivore diet is taking up the slack. This diet has become popular with many influencers promoting it, although most of them have little or no health training. The carnivore diet is exactly as it sounds: all meat, all the time. No plants whatsoever. Eggs and some dairy are allowed, but many promoters talk about eating only steaks. This diet has *zero* long-term studies other than anecdotal accounts, which means there's neither any hard science on how to set it up properly nor long-term studies to see how the body copes with running on nothing but meat. Following the diet for an extended period may have serious consequences that haven't been discovered yet. Be wary with this one—very, very wary.

Five Hallmarks of a Fad Diet

When you review dieting history, it's easy to spot (and, frankly, mock) a fad, but it can be much harder to spot the fad diets when they first arrive and promise many things. You might be eager to buy in to these diets as easy solutions to all of your health problems (especially any weight issues), so it can be hard to resist jumping on the bandwagon.

Fad diets have a few key characteristics. Keep the following five traits in mind anytime a hot new diet blows into town, and steer clear of all of the stress and frustration of trying something that goes against what your body wants.

1. Fad diets promise an easy, quick fix that seems almost too good to be true.

If the promoters of a diet say things like, "drop 10 pounds or more in two weeks," or, "reverse all of your health conditions overnight," then run far, far away. Before you embark on a crash fad diet, you need to know one crucial thing: Fast weight loss is almost always water weight.

Low-carb diets trigger a release of water, but the moment a little bit of something sweet passes your lips, all of that water will come right back. (And that's good; you were probably dehydrated on a cellular level without that water.)

If the weight loss isn't water weight, then it's usually due to muscle loss. Real fat loss takes some time. Losing muscle means your metabolism might slow down, and you're guaranteed to gain back that lost muscle as fat unless you're doing heavy muscle training.

Rapid weight loss also increases the hunger hormone ghrelin, which can make your hunger seem insatiable. Boo! Keep your muscle and water where it is. Slow and steady permanent weight loss is the healthiest way.

2. Fad diets promote a simple solution to a complex problem, usually vilifying some type of food many people regularly consume.

As you already know, macronutrients are all *essential* for your body to work correctly. In the low-fat 1980s, dieters didn't receive enough essential fats to regulate inflammation. They also didn't have enough fat to balance out all of the sugar and refined carbs that had been added to low-fat food to make it taste better. The result was higher rates of obesity and heart disease, two conditions the low-fat diet was supposed to protect people from.

If you follow a low-carb plan, your body is missing out on the primary macronutrient that gives it energy. Although some people can do okay with few carbs, other people experience huge sugar binges because they have particularly carb-lovin' bodies. (I fit into this category.) Plus, your body needs carbohydrates for hormone production, something that's especially important for women during perimenopause. I've found its women in their forties and fifties who are most commonly on a low-carb diet to stave off any hormone-induced weight gain, but that plan can cause a whole host of other problems.

3. Fad diets offer a one-size-fits-all solution that will create incredibly fast results.

You might think that the days of meal replacement shakes from the 1980s and 1990s are over, but the idea of drinking a shake for two meals each day is still alive and well. New meal replacement products are, for the most part, better quality than what was offered thirty years ago, but the idea is the same. Drinking meal replacement shakes can trigger weight loss for a while (as any super low-calorie diet will), but no one can live for the rest of their lives this way. When you give up on the plan, whatever weight you lost comes right back. Think of it as boomerang weight loss.

4. Fad diets promote a "new" discovery of the body's chemistry—something no one realized in the past.

A frequent telltale sign of a fad diet is that the promoters claim to have discovered a new understanding of human biology—like when those who evangelize the ketogenic diet claimed that *this* is the newly discovered perfect diet of the future.

Pretending that human biology doesn't exist or that someone has discovered a new truth to human biology is a classic attribute with fad diets. So far, the claims have always been dead wrong. Remember the low-/no-fat diet of the 1980s? It caused a spike in obesity and heart disease rates that was an unexpected shock to all of the low-fat diet experts; it took thirty years to figure that out. We don't yet know what shunning carbs will do to overall health, but within a decade or so, we'll have some idea, and people will have moved on to another "discovery."

5. Fad diets promote low daily calorie intake.

Your body's metabolism is like a furnace that's powered by the food you eat. If you stoke the fire regularly, then it burns brightly. However, if you regularly limit how much food you eat (eating less than 1,500 calories per day), then your inner furnace has to learn how to function with less fuel. Your body responds in the only way it can: It dims the fire and slows down your whole system. Restrictive diets aren't healthy diets!

Research has found that low-calorie diets slow your metabolism while you're following the plan and even when you stop. Some studies have found that a low-calorie diet can cause your body to burn up to 23 percent fewer calories in a day! Yikes! When your metabolism makes that kind of shift, your body now needs one-quarter less food that it previously did. Unfortunately, low-calorie diets tend to make you feel hungry, so eating less food is really hard to accomplish.

Wrapping It All Up

Fad diets lead to enormous food guilt and a lot of *shoulds.* "I should be able to eat less. I shouldn't be so hungry all the time. I should be able to control my eating better." No, you shouldn't because you *can't!* It's impossible when your body works against those efforts!

Your body loves you exactly as you are right now and gets really worried and stressed out if you follow a low-calorie diet. The slowing down of your metabolism and your increased appetite is your body's way of finding balance. The fad diet was the problem—NOT YOU! You didn't do anything wrong, other than follow some dieting advice with the very best of intentions.

The weight-loss industry is a $150 billion industry, and the profitability is what drives the incredibly unhealthy dieting culture. The dieting culture doesn't want you to know how to eat for yourself because it wants you to be reliant on its ever-changing campaign of "perfect" dieting ideas. You can walk off the dieting treadmill anytime, though—including right now.

Now that you know the red flags of a fad diet, you'll find it easier to ignore them until they fizzle out. I think it's important that we also recognize how many problematic dieting ideas have burrowed deep into our minds to make it hard to recognize the difference between *healthy eating* and *dieting.* In the next chapter, I peel apart dieting culture so you can see that it's profit, not health, that drives this industry.

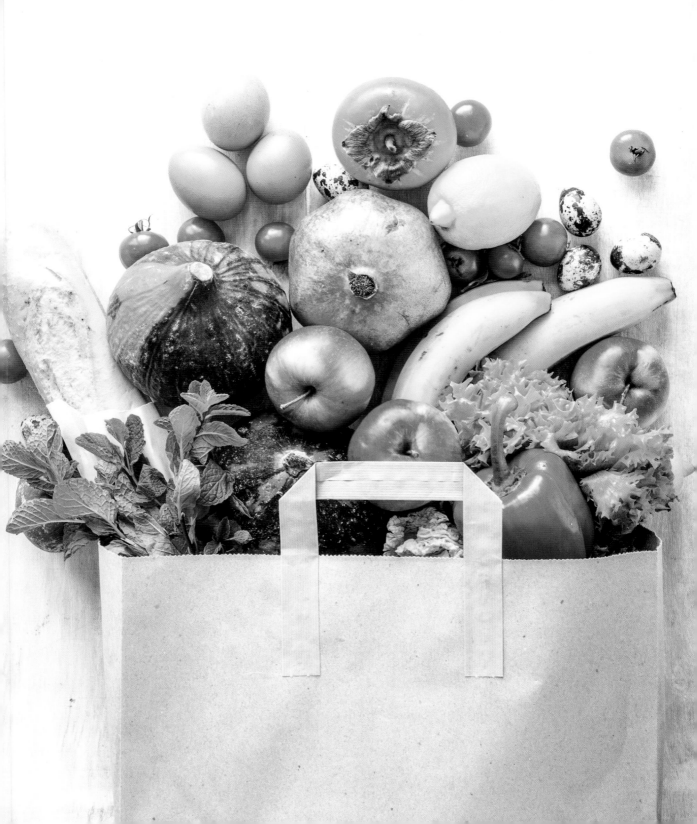

chapter

06

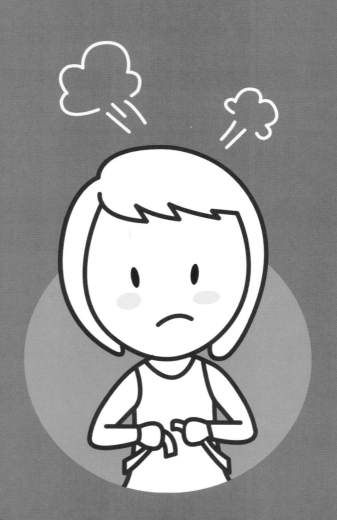

WHY DIETS DON'T WORK

Your body really wants you to be healthy, happy, and full of energy, and that's something that can happen in a wonderful (and delicious) way!

However, in our weight-obsessed, Insta-filtered society, it can be so hard to keep your focus on better health rather than the promises of weight-loss fads. I'd argue—quite adamantly—that better health is what you should focus on. Weight loss is a nice side effect of a healthier diet and lifestyle, but when people focus only on weight loss and go on a "diet," then they're usually worse off than before. It's an unfortunate truth.

When researchers followed up on participants from thirty-one different weight-loss studies, they found that most participants would have been better off if they hadn't dieted at all. Eighty to ninety-five percent of dieters will gain back everything they've lost, making most diets a very futile effort. It isn't better for serial dieters; in a study that followed 19,000 men, the best indicator that a participant would gain weight back was that he'd been on a diet before participating in the study.

Ugh, am I right? For years, you've heard that going on a diet is the only way to be healthier and lose weight. In truth, though, diets are a relatively quick fix for a long-term problem. You may feel better or lose weight for a while, but a while doesn't equal forever.

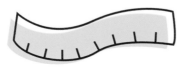

In this chapter, I'll be taking you on a trip through the political and financial motivations of the dieting industry. You'll see that even the most basic measurement of your weight, the BMI, has been influenced by the dieting industry. Buckle up; it's going to be a bumpy ride!

Why Fad Diets Fail

Why is it that after decades of research and more than 150 years of experts giving weight-loss advice, most people who embark on a diet fail? (In this case, I'm defining *failure* as "didn't lose any weight" or "gained the weight back.") Why haven't we figured this out yet?

The promise of diet fads is that people can eat (almost) anything they want as long as they kick one "bad," vilified macronutrient to the curb. Then the pounds will just melt away. Many of these diets also proclaim that people can easily follow them for as long as necessary—forever even! *Suuuuuure.* That'll work. If that was possible, or if any of these diets worked in the long run, people would follow them for years and years after the diets are first introduced. It's really hard to find someone who sticks with a fad diet for longer than a few months.

The vilification of one macronutrient means you don't have access to many foods. If you follow a low-fat diet, you can't have chips and fatty meats. If you follow a low-carb diet, you're denied sugary foods. Restrictive diets make it hard to eat in restaurants or enjoy a meal at a friend's house, and they also make mindless snacking really difficult. Mindless eating can make up a huge portion of your diet, and by eliminating snacks, you're cutting calories. So, diets that cut out one macronutrient are really just a reinvention of the old 1970s way of dieting, which is to eat less and exercise more—more calories out than calories in.

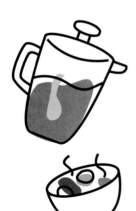

Calories In Versus Calories Out Doesn't Work

Well, calories in versus calories out does work, but it's a lot more complicated than it seems. The idea of fewer calories in and more calories out is just too simplistic because there are so many other factors that influence weight, like stress, sleep quality, gut bacteria, and your body's nutrient balance.

What is a calorie anyhow? A calorie is the amount of heat needed to raise the temperature of 1 kilogram of water by 1 degree Celsius. How could this measurement relate to the complicated way food interacts with your body? That concept is hard to apply in real life, especially when scientists are always learning new things about how bodies extract energy from food, including that raw food provides less energy than cooked food.

The human body has a fantastic protective mechanism that came about when food was scarce. It's from a time when humans had to work diligently to get food, so maintaining a healthy body weight was a vital job of metabolism.

It's only been a short period since food has become amazingly abundant and easy to procure; with a quick phone call, you can have a full feast delivered to your door. The human body hasn't adapted to this sort of abundance yet, and it still thinks that food is hard to come by. Another issue is that your body assumes that your current weight is your ideal weight, even if you have a different idea. When you go on a very calorie-restrictive diet and begin to lose weight, your body goes into panic mode and tries to stop the madness because it believes the lack of calories is a sign that you're dealing with a famine.

When you start to restrict calories, the first thing your body does is to *sloooooow doooooown*. Your body slows your metabolism, reduces your energy level, and eliminates any extra energy output. Studies have shown that people burn a surprising amount of energy by fidgeting, but other studies have uncovered that people fidget a lot less when they eat less. Slowing down the body to conserve energy when there's a perceived famine is an important survival mechanism; this conservation of energy may have played a significant role in human survival. For some, this survival mechanism can trigger a weight-loss plateau; for others, it can prevent any weight loss from the get-go. Unfortunately, when your metabolism has slowed, it's very easy for you to regain weight.

A study that followed winners of *The Biggest Loser* showcases this very annoying issue. When the participants began the show, they all had normal metabolisms for their size and a normal resting metabolism (the amount of energy you burn when you're sitting on the couch, resting). After the participants had lost a lot of weight, their resting metabolisms had slowed dramatically. Sadly, their metabolisms didn't recover even when the scale started to creep back up. One winner, Danny Cahill, had such a dramatic slowdown of his metabolism that to maintain his weight at 295 pounds, he needed to eat 800 calories less per day than another person his size would have needed to eat. The rapid weight loss caused by fad diets can cause these terrible long-term problems.

Other Dieting Problems

A few years ago, I worked with a woman who had put herself on a low-carb, high-protein diet that was also very low in calories. She was determined to drop some weight quickly, so she was also going to the gym almost every day. Salads and protein were the main staples in her diet, but she wasn't losing any weight. I saw her over a few sessions, and I was surprised that her body wasn't desperately craving carbohydrates. All of the energy she was burning at the gym needed a steady supply of glucose, and salad greens aren't usually good enough. She reported that she wasn't craving anything.

However, it wasn't long before she started having a big craving. Every few days, her body would scream for a favorite food: marshmallows. Eventually, she gave in. Because she had denied herself for so long, her willpower was low, and she *really* gave in. Like clockwork, she would eat an entire bag of marshmallows every three days. I don't believe that this indulgence

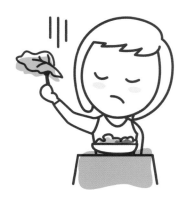

was a sign of weakness; it's just that her diet was wildly out of balance for her body, and one's body always wins. Her body found a way to get the energy it was looking for.

Your body doesn't like it when you eliminate macronutrients. Have you ever had a craving that was so strong that it was all you could think about? Did it sit at the back of your mind until you finally satisfied it? Yup. Me, too. I think it's a universal human experience. This craving is your body trying to satisfy its need for something. Sometimes the craving is purely emotional; your body wants you to feel a bit of pleasure. Usually, though, your body wants something that food can provide. It might be some extra salt (a chip craving) or magnesium (a chocolate craving) or some carbs/starch (a sweet craving).

When your body wants something, it *always* wins. The feeling can seem pretty sinister, but it's just about balance. Say you're following a protein/veggie/low-carb style of diet. You feel terrific, and your energy is steady, but, man! Those cookies (or whatever sweet loveliness you like) look delicious! You can say no over and over again, but eventually, you'll be too tired to refuse one more time. Those cookies are so enticing, you'll (guiltily) indulge—maybe with more than one (maybe even the whole package).

I can't stress enough that this "giving in" isn't due to a lack of willpower. (After all, you needed *tons* of willpower to say "no" so many times.) It's not (usually) emotional eating, either. Instead, it was your body asking for something, and your body was victorious. It got what it was looking for. When you restrict food or eliminate whole macronutrients, your body isn't happy, and eventually, it'll be triumphant. It always is.

Low thyroid function and adrenal fatigue (aka burnout or chronic exhaustion; read more in Chapter 10) can also stop any weight loss in its tracks. If you're concerned your thyroid might be a problem, the first thing to do is to have your thyroid levels checked. Your doctor can order a test, and it's a good thing to check regularly. Having your thyroid tested is especially important if you feel cold, slow, or tired; are losing hair; or have a bad case of the blahs.

Adrenal glands also get tired pretty darn quickly if you try to maintain a go-go-go lifestyle. When your stress level is high, so is your cortisol, which gives you tons of energy and helps you feel good until you finally sit down and crash. Eventually, your adrenals get worn out, and you start dealing with low cortisol levels.

Subclinical low cortisol can feel like a chronic state of exhaustion. You're tired all day long, and you lose all of your drive, motivation, and "I CAN DO THIS!" attitude. Higher cortisol can add 10 to 20 pounds (or more) of weight around your waist, and lower levels of cortisol can make that weight unbelievably stubborn. Usually, it won't move until your adrenals are happier. Thyroid issues usually occur after your adrenals have been overworked for a long time, so these two issues frequently come together.

Your microbiome also plays a role in how much energy you extract from the food you eat. Two people can eat identical meals, but each will absorb a different amount of energy depending on their gut bacteria. Research has found that people usually extract more energy from food when the gut bacteria community is weak (this may depend on the strains that are left). They've found that people with a low diversity of bacteria in their guts have slower metabolisms and have a higher risk of obesity.

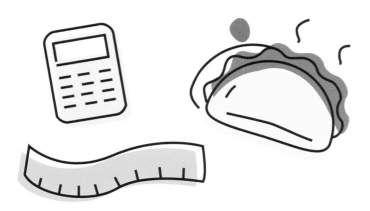

The American Gut Project, the largest ever crowd-sourced study (people have literally sent their poop to the researchers), has found that the diversity of the diet equals the diversity of the gut bacteria. Also, more plant-based fiber means a more robust inner ecosystem. If you spend your day eating the same low-fiber foods, like white bread, sugary muffins, meat, and dairy, then you'll have a weaker community of gut bacteria than someone who eats a lot of veggies, and this lack of diversity may slow your metabolism. Many fad diets, especially the super low-carb diets, can lower gut bacteria diversity due to the lack of plant-based fiber.

Lastly, calorie counts on Nutrition Facts labels might be wildly incorrect. You can be a diligent calorie counter and exercise tracker, but your scale might not budge simply because your calorie count might be as much as 20 percent off! The FDA allows for as much as 20 percent inaccuracies on that pesky Nutrition Facts label.

So, can we agree that this calorie-counting thing is full of problems?

Even the BMI Scale Is a Tad Problematic

What if I said that the Body Mass Index (BMI) scale used by most doctors to determine whether you're overweight was highly influenced by the weight-loss industry? You'd be pretty furious—am I right?

The BMI has become a healthcare standard for determining what's a healthy weight and what's considered overweight or obese. Both height and weight are factors, and for many people, the BMI number sits at the top of the doctor's medical chart.

In 1998, approximately 29 million Americans became over-weight overnight, without having gained a pound, when a panel of experts at the National Institutes of Health (NIH) decided to shift the BMI overweight category from 27.5 to 25. In his book *Fat Politics*, author J. Eric Oliver says that this decision was highly influenced by the dieting industry. According to Oliver, the chairman of the committee had strong ties to several manufacturers of diet drugs and Weight Watchers.

I bet the dieting industry loved the new guidelines!

Not all of the members of the NIH committee agreed with this decision. Obesity researcher Judy Stern was an outspoken critic of these new changes and the only member of the committee who voted against it. Stern was against making this change because she felt the decision was based on misquoted data, flawed science, and industry influence. Fifteen years later, a new meta-analysis agreed with Stern. The meta-analysis looked at ninety-seven studies involving three million people and found that people in the overweight category actually had a 6 percent lower risk of death than those in the healthy weight category.

So, you might be perfectly healthy just as you are, even if your BMI is a bit higher than your doctor would like.

These are the kinds of industry tricks that are found throughout dieting culture. The dieting industry has convinced people to cut calories, but the food industry pushes people to eat more. Your failures feel personal when in reality they're just inevitable. Every day you're bombarded by commercials, print ads, and billboards that are trying to lure you into eating more and more of food manufacturers' products. I find that I get hungry anytime I watch TV commercials, even if I've just eaten. The repetitive commercials showcasing gooey pizza, sweet delights, and perfectly styled hamburgers make my mouth water. No wonder we collectively have weight issues; we're only human. I believe that canceling my cable subscription played a big role in my ability to achieve a healthy life; I'm no longer tempted by those commercials!

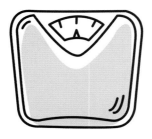

Wrapping It All Up

I hope this chapter has given you a sense of why dieting culture is messed up and helped you understand that the food industry and government have falsely set the parameters around what is considered healthy and acceptable.

By moving away from manufactured food products and into whole food, you can achieve real health, and the by-product of whole-food eating is frequently the weight loss you've been looking for.

In Part 3, I bring you back to your body as I take you through the steps you need to take in order to walk away from the dieting mentality and learn your body's language. This is where real undieting begins.

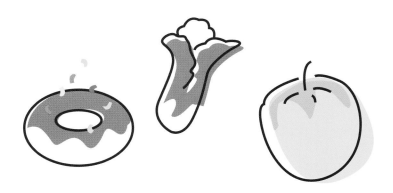

PART 3

BODY LANGUAGE

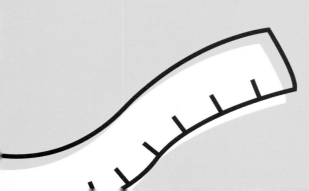

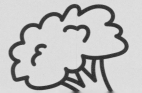

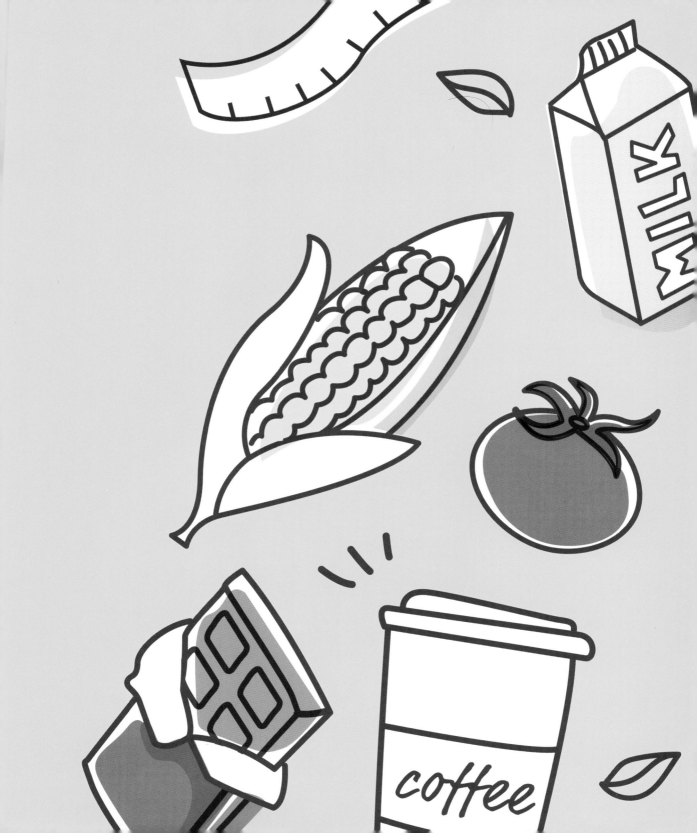

chapter

07

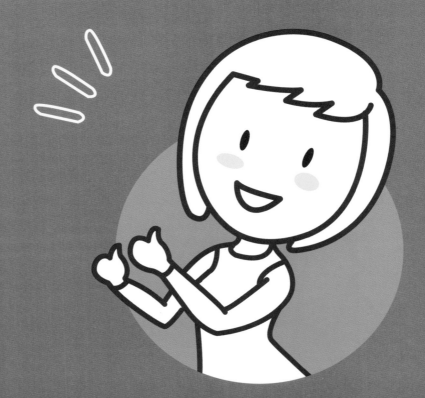

YOUR BODY'S TOOL KIT

It's time for the good stuff: how to understand your body's language and how to use that knowledge to find a way of eating that's perfect for you. This part of the book is a guide for learning your body's language and reframing your eating habits. Each of the following chapters takes you through a different way to look at your symptoms and guides you through the steps to find balance.

Take each step one at a time. You can go through them in the order I've listed them, or you can start with the step that seems most interesting to you. Each step will take you further away from fad dieting culture and toward your inner wisdom. Your body wants to be heard, but you need to understand what it's saying. Let's dive in!

Your Body Always Wins—and That's a Good Thing

Being on a diet is a struggle for anyone. Sometimes you may find you can go weeks or even months (or sometimes years) on a diet without a hint of trouble, but eventually, the struggle will start. It's not a sign of weakness or a lack of willpower; it's just an inevitability of being human.

The struggle is a sign that your body wants a change. Whatever you've been doing may have been fine last week or last month, but it's sure as heck not okay now. The sign could manifest as a huge craving that's hard to say no to or an old habit that creeps back into your life. I've seen this struggle be everything from indulging in a night of junk food to spending a full year eating everything that had been missing from a diet.

The frustrating pattern I've seen over and over again is that the longer you've deprived yourself of something you love, the longer it'll take to get back to a healthy diet after you've fallen off the wagon. Basically, the more willpower you have, the greater the chance that you'll have a very long eating detour.

When you take a detour, your body isn't trying to sabotage you and move you away from health; it's just trying to find balance. It's not a surprise that your body might scream for sugar anytime you deprive it of everything sweet. There's a wonderful silver lining here, though: Instead of depriving yourself of everything you love that doesn't fit inside the "healthy" box, you can look at your cravings as a request for balance.

It's time to replace willpower with curiosity!

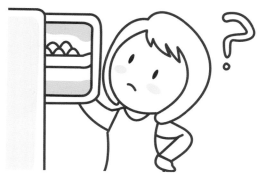

Falling off the Wagon: The Best Way to Secure a Healthy Change

Before I became a nutritionist, I assumed that health coaches and nutritionists were all great at living perfectly healthy lives. I looked at the ease in which they lived their healthy lifestyles and thought that they had worked out all of the kinks and ate a beautiful diet every single day. Then I became a nutritionist and realized that I'm human—and so is every other nutritionist. We're all beautifully imperfect humans.

I also discovered that the moments of imperfection are when I learn the most about healthy eating. Every time I move away from my healthy habits, I learn something new about my body.

For example, last fall, I took advantage of the time change to get back to an earlier bedtime. I love going to be bed early, and I feel best when I'm in the dark by 10:00 p.m. The preceding summer, my bedtime had started to push to 10:30 or 11:00 p.m., and I wanted to get back to my early bedtime habit. Enough was enough, and when it was the night to "fall back" because of the time change, I dutifully got ready for bed at 9:30 p.m. I felt the difference immediately.

Later that same week, my partner (a musician) had a gig on a weeknight, and I wanted to go. His gig wasn't over until after 10:00 p.m., so I didn't get in bed until after 11:00, well past my newly minted early bedtime. But schedule fluctuations are part of real life, and my healthy lifestyle needs to work inside real life. If it doesn't, well, it's not going to work in the long term, is it?

Unsurprisingly, I woke up the next morning feeling super-duper tired. In that moment of sleepiness, I had two choices: I could berate myself and feel guilty for "falling off" my new healthy habit, or I could be curious about it.

The thing I hate about dieting or other health commitments that have gone sideways is the guilt people have been conditioned to feel whenever their actions don't perfectly measure up against healthy habits. It's impossible to learn from these moments if you're swimming in guilt. It's too easy to blame yourself instead of noticing what happened, which was real life. Real life always happens; you can count on it. I choose to embrace real life, so on that morning, I chose to be curious about how I felt instead of wallowing in guilt.

I lay in bed and really examined the difference between how I felt on the morning after a 10:00 p.m. bedtime versus how I felt on the morning after going to bed just one hour later.

I didn't like it. I didn't like the sleepiness or the cobwebs I had to knock out of my brain. It was at that moment that I quickly and easily recommitted to my earlier bedtime. I even looked forward to going to bed early that night. Using a compassionate mindset when confronting challenges to your healthy routines can make all the difference sometimes.

This approach of being curious when my healthy habits slip began when I first started working one on one with clients. I noticed a common pattern; my clients would come to the second appointment feeling fantastic. They were full of energy and vitality, and they were full-on committed to the changes we were making.

Between the second and third appointments, though, life would happen. My clients would come to the third appointment dripping in guilt. They would sit down, give me a guilt-ridden look, and say, "You're going to be so disappointed in me. I almost canceled this appointment. I was away last weekend and ate a ton of junk food."

They'd wait for me to add to their guilt, but that's not how I roll. Instead, I would ask, "So, how do you feel?" The answers were usually very similar to mine on that sleepy morning: tired, foggy, and miserable. Then I'd ask, "What are you craving now?"

The answer was always the same, "VEGETABLES! I never thought I'd ever crave vegetables, but that's all I want!"

This example demonstrates the power of staying curious. With curiosity, you can learn so much when real life happens and gets in your way. Curiosity dissolves guilt on the spot, and it allows you to see what's really going on. When your healthy habits slip, you get an opportunity to reflect on how much better you felt before the slip. It gives you a valuable before-and-after view! I quickly fell in love with the common appointment #3 slip-up. It became a powerful tool for my tool kit.

Remember, undieting means that you don't "fall off the wagon" because you were never on a wagon to start with. Instead, you begin by adding healthy food and let it squish out some less-than-stellar food. When your habit slips a bit, be curious. Examine how that slip feels.

Stay curious, and you'll quickly find yourself gravitating toward healthier habits with ease. And ease is powerful. Ease is joyous. Ease is beautiful.

Without a Structure to Follow, What Do I Do?

Undieting would be so much more straightforward with a meal plan, right? A guide to follow or exact instructions to go by so you know you're doing everything correctly. But undieting really isn't that difficult when you embrace a few simple guidelines.

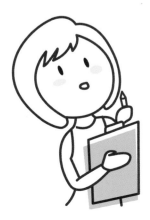

In my first few years as a nutritionist, many of my clients asked me for a meal plan. Making meal plans for other people was always a frustrating chore. I know what a healthy meal plan looks like, and I know what I like to eat, but it was impossible to leap inside other people's heads to figure out what they'd enjoy. I did it, though; I made a meal plan for every client who asked me for one. I labored and stressed over them, and I hated every second of it. It was, without question, my least favorite part of my work. Otherwise, I loved what I did.

It wasn't long before I noticed a pattern. No one—and I mean *not one person*—followed any of the meal plans I toiled over so diligently. I didn't blame them; I wouldn't have followed them either. Meal plans turn healthy eating into a job, and they steal pleasure and enjoyment from eating.

If you follow a structure or a plan too rigidly, you lose out on pleasure. The chore of following a meal plan is the opposite of pleasure. You stop listening to your body's guidance because you're trying to ignore your cravings and wants. Simply put, meal plans don't respect your body's wisdom, and following a meal plan or a structured diet program is a short-term solution. Staying on course takes loads and loads of willpower, and you're left where you started as soon as your willpower runs out. Instead, there's a different way—one that embraces pleasurable eating and requires almost no willpower.

GIVE YOUR BRAIN A NEW JOB

Your brain loves structure and meal plans, but your body wants what it wants. Your brain loves to find solutions, and your body already knows what it needs. If your brain is too loud and takes over, you miss out on much of your body's innate wisdom, and you can find yourself struggling to make changes. Struggle is a sign that your brain is trying to be in charge.

Try flipping things around and giving your brain a new job. Instead of being in charge of figuring out your health "problem," let your body do that while your brain works on interpreting your body's language. Your brain loves to work; it just needs some guidance.

Making this change can be hard to do if you've spent time inside the dieting culture. If you've ever strictly followed a diet, meal plan, or food plan, then your brain is used to being in charge of your health. It can be hard to start trusting your body because it can send signals that you perceive to be unhealthy, like "I want cookies!" or "Gimme some chips!"

Your body wants to be healthier, too, but it just may not be asking for the right food. Its request for cookies might be a request for some slow-burning starchy food (like sweet potatoes), but it just doesn't know it yet because it hasn't enjoyed them (or has, but guilty feelings negated those good feelings). Similarly, your body's request for chips might be a request for more food with sea salt.

Learning the language of your body can be a tough job, but it's the perfect challenge for your brain. It allows your brain to do what it's good at—thinking. Then you can let your body do what it's good at—feeling and staying balanced. Your brain and your body make a great team as soon as they're doing their correct jobs. The trick is this:

Let your body feel the cravings. Then let your brain figure out the right food to combat those cravings in the healthiest way.

FIND YOUR MOTIVATION

You need motivation to make even the smallest change, and the best motivators are emotion based.

The human brain has a talent for identifying motivations, like being healthier, losing weight, or getting in better shape. But the body doesn't care about those rational ideas because it speaks in emotion. When you find a motivation that speaks to your body, then it's easier to stay motivated even when you're moving through your day on autopilot. In other words, if your motivation is something rational and unemotional like *getting in better shape*, it can be hard to stop yourself from automatically grabbing that cookie on the counter. Instead, if your motivation is emotional—*I want to keep up with my peers/kids/grandkids*—then you have a better chance of staying present enough to forgo that cookie.

Your body needs you to feel the motivation—not just think about it. Close your eyes and think about what it will be like when your body starts to feel better, like when you have enough energy to play with your kids or grandkids all afternoon. Or when you can run a 5k. Or when you have enough energy to get to the end of the day without being completely out of juice.

Find your emotional motivation and embrace it.

SHRINK THE CHANGE

The best chance of making a permanent change is when you feel 95 percent confident that you can do it. Biting off more than you can chew can lead to a lot of frustration and disappointment, and I've seen over and over again that real change can happen surprisingly quickly with a bunch of tiny, easy changes.

Big confidence creates big wins, which gives you even more confidence so you can keep going. Don't worry about looking for a challenge; life is already challenging enough. Instead, shrink the change you make until it's so easy you feel just about 100 percent confident you can knock it out of the park.

THE MAGIC OF ADDING HEALTHY FOODS

If there's one thing I want you to remember it's this: always add healthy foods before removing anything.

There are so many nutrition experts who warn about dangers like gluten, dairy, sugar, and processed food. For some people who have certain health conditions, it might be a good idea to remove these foods for a period. However—I can't stress this enough—*don't* remove anything until you've added a bunch of other healthy food first.

You want to know why? When you remove something, you're left with a giant hole in your diet that needs to be filled. Say you remove gluten but usually start your day with toast and then have a sandwich for lunch. By removing gluten, you now have to find a new breakfast *and* a new option for lunch, even if that just means finding a gluten-free bread you like. If you don't quickly find new options for the foods you've removed, then you're apt to fill that hole in your diet with a bunch of the old gluten-filled food.

Instead, add a bunch of new foods and let those items squish out the less-than-fabulous food. Try out some new breakfasts to see how they feel. Add some more servings of fruit and veggies, try out some new vegetarian meals, and experiment with some new grains like quinoa or buckwheat.

Adding new food first is a powerful way to make healthy changes easily. It's like magic.

Wrapping It All Up

As your guide on your journey to better health through undieting, I need to give you some hard truths.

You're going to make many wonderful changes to and for your body when you eat a healthier diet. You'll feel healthier and have more energy. Your skin will glow, and your eyes will brighten (you can literally be bright-eyed and bushy-tailed). You can be stronger and more resilient, and you'll have less inflammation and pain. And you can feel SO much better.

Will you lose weight? Probably. But maybe not.

Weight loss is often a pleasant side effect of a healthier, more balanced diet. But other factors are playing out in your body, and for some people, the scale doesn't budge easily. Your body loves you exactly as you are right now and gets worried if you start to lose too much weight. As I mentioned earlier in the book, if your food intake drops, your body wonders if there's a famine and slows down your metabolism to put the brakes on your weight loss.

I want to encourage you to eat a healthier diet regardless of whether it moves the scale because feeling better is just so marvelous! You need to know that you're extraordinary exactly as you are.

My friend Wendy Goudie is an incredible belly-dancer and teacher in Penticton, British Columbia. Through dance, she promotes loving one's body and showcasing beautiful curves. She would encourage everyone to hike up their shirts and show their bellies while dancing, but, especially at the beginning, it can be hard to show off your belly while dancing in front of a mirror.

I took a few beginner classes with Wendy, and I'll always remember her gentle encouragement. She would tell the class that belly dancing is a wonderful way to make peace with your stomach and curves and that most women fall in love with their bellies in dance and miss them once they've transformed.

Through the undieting process, as you learn the language and genius of your body, I encourage you to fall in love with your body, belly, and curves too. You might just miss them when they're gone.

In the next chapters, I share the steps for listening to your body, walking away from diet culture, and reframing your eating habits. You can work through the process in the order that I've laid it out, or you can skip around to do it in whatever way seems best for you:

- Finding out what your cravings mean

- Figuring out what your digestion is telling you

- Regaining your energy

- Maximizing pleasure and enjoyment

And remember the mantra: Your body always wins. You just need to figure out what your body is trying to say!

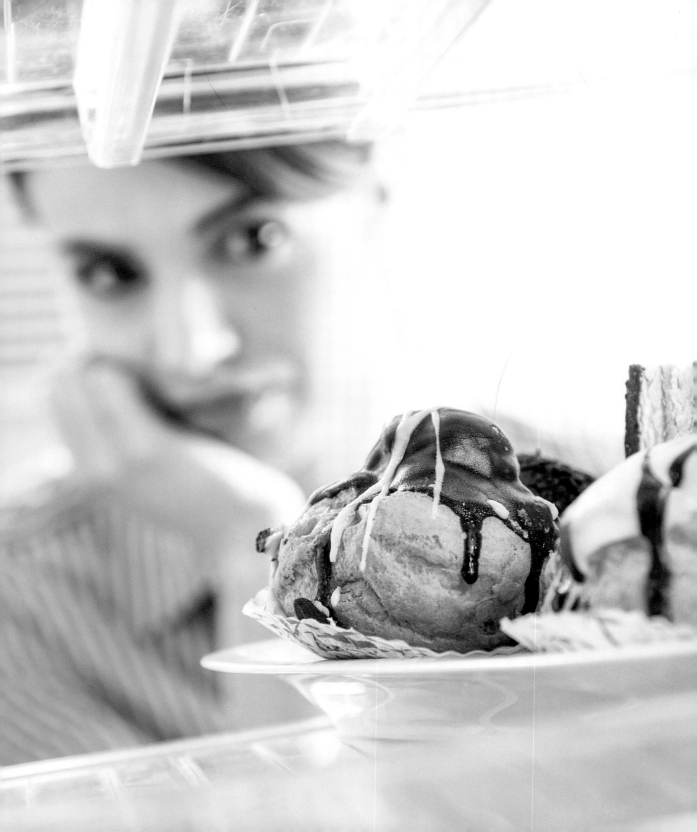

WHAT ARE YOUR CRAVINGS TELLING YOU?

I've heard it so many times: "A healthy diet would be so easy if I didn't love chocolate so much." Or potato chips. Or pastries. Or anything delectable.

Food cravings are an intense desire for food. Remember that word: *intense*. It's the intensity of a craving that makes saying "no" so hard to do, no matter how determined you are. You can use every ounce of willpower you have, but eventually, a moment will come when your willpower runs out, and you'll indulge. Then, with that lovely, delectable food comes feelings of guilt and weakness and sometimes shame. Instead of enjoying this food you love, you're dripping in regret.

But it doesn't have to be that way! When your body wants something so badly that you crave it, a reason is usually behind that craving. When you understand why you're craving something, all of the guilty feelings disappear like magic.

So, look at this situation a bit differently. Instead of seeing cravings as something to power through, try listening to them and looking for the subtle clues your body is trying to give you.

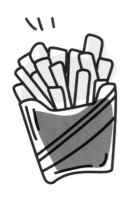

Cravings Defined

What, when, and why you crave food tells you a lot about nutritional imbalances, blood sugar imbalances, and deficiencies. Without these cravings, my job as a nutritionist would be much harder. Your cravings are a valuable guide to your body's unique language.

Also, cravings are a wonderful part of being human. Imagine life without that first bite of chocolate cake or the melting of a croissant on the tongue. This kind of pleasure is so sublime!

Cravings are one of the reasons why following a set diet plan simply doesn't work in the long run. You can't possibly have enough willpower to say no to your favorite food forever. It would be like holding a 5-pound weight over your head for days; eventually, you're going to drop it. I've found that the longer you say no to a particular food, the more of it you'll eat once your willpower runs out. I've watched it happen time and time again, and I've lived it myself.

In my mid-twenties, I realized that a mild dairy sensitivity was affecting my breathing. I was a music student, studying the flute, and I was ready to do anything if it meant I could reliably breathe during rehearsals. The problem was that everything I ate had dairy in it. I was determined, though, and I honestly felt a lot better when I didn't have any dairy.

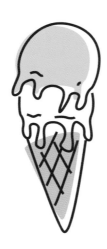

It took every ounce of willpower I had to get through each day. My diet was terrible, and all of my favorite processed foods included dairy. Grocery shopping was a miserable experience because I didn't know what to buy. Going to restaurants was a trial. To get by, I ate the same boxed nondairy macaroni for lunch and dinner every single day. I was miserable, even though I felt a lot better physically.

I went to a party during this time, and an acquaintance was sitting beside me, eating ice cream. It wasn't even a flavor of ice cream I liked, but I knew she was eating something I couldn't have. I sat beside this woman I barely knew and seethed. All I could think was, "How *dare* she eat ice cream in front of me? Doesn't she know what I'm going through? Doesn't she realize how hard this is for me?!"

Yes, my reaction was unreasonable, but that was precisely how I felt at the time.

Saying no to a craving over and over again is impossible because your body will eventually get what it wants. Your body always wins.

My first dairy-free experiment lasted four miserable months and ended with my first hour-long solo recital. The day after my recital, I enjoyed a big plate of nachos, and I continued my dairy binge for the next four years. It didn't matter to me that my breathing had become difficult again or that my nose was constantly stuffy. All that mattered was that I had access to unlimited amounts of cheese, yogurt, and ice cream.

Delicious, *delicious* ice cream.

Today, I've had minimal dairy in my diet for about twelve years. I've been successful with my second attempt to have a dairy-free diet because I've never deprived myself of it. I can have it anytime I want, and I'll enjoy some dairy if I'm really craving it. (I don't have a deadly allergy—just a sensitivity.)

My almost-dairy-free life came about in the same way as my healthy diet, slowly and step by step. One by one, I replaced my favorite dairy foods with something that I liked just as much. Cheese on my salad became toasted almonds. Cheese on my sandwich became avocado. I found an alternative recipe for Parmesan made from cashews and nutritional yeast that made my taste buds very happy. I switched to coconut milk on my cereal, and I was thrilled when coconut and cashew milk ice creams came onto the market.

Today, I usually can recognize a craving quickly, which allows me to analyze what the craving means to my body so I can consciously make a healthy and satisfying choice.

I always stay curious about my cravings; what is it that my body is looking for? If I really want cheese, then I'll have some and enjoy every bite. Usually, though, I have so many other delicious alternatives that I can satisfy my craving with a dairy-free option. Now I even prefer dairy-free ice cream over regular ice cream, but I will indulge in the real thing if I'm at a great ice cream shop, such as The Opinicon in Ontario, Canada's cottage country. Heck, I am human, after all.

This gentleness I offer myself has helped me ease dairy out of my diet. Notice the word *ease*. By staying engaged in my cravings, I have been able to learn more about what my body is looking for. When I crave anything, I consciously choose to eat it, and I enjoy every bite, which enables me to deeply feel what it means to my body.

Cravings: Your Body's Whispered Requests

I believe that every craving is a request from your body for something. Maybe you're missing a mineral, or maybe you're dealing with an imbalance that you haven't recognized, such as lots of stress or chronic inflammation. By learning what your body is looking for, your cravings become gentler, easier, and less demanding.

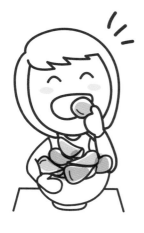

Over the years, I've worked with thousands of people, and I've noticed many similarities in their cravings. These are anecdotal connections, but they seem to hold lots of truth. Your cravings may fit nicely into the categories I've used in this chapter, or you may need to dig further and carry out more detective work to find connections and solutions that are right for you. When you look at your cravings as the language of your body, they become less frustrating, and that allows you to save your willpower. There are many better uses of willpower than denying yourself food all day. Understanding your body is so liberating!

In the following sections, I mostly connect cravings to nutrients that your body might be looking for, but you should also keep in mind that what your body might be connecting to is a memory of comfort or pleasure. For example, my favorite food as a kid was salt and vinegar potato chips (a very Canadian flavor), and I watched a lot of TV. Now, in adulthood, when I'm feeling overwhelmed, all I want to do is eat salt and vinegar chips and watch a TV show that's an old favorite. The theme song of the show mixed with the crunch of the chips relaxes me, and it brings me some comfort that offsets my chaotic feelings. In those moments, my body isn't looking for more salt or potatoes; it's just looking for comfort.

Keep that in mind as you go through the following sections. Once you've read through all of Part 3, you'll be better able to assess whether your body is looking for nutrients or comfort. In the meantime, just keep paying attention to your feelings. Knowing the physical causes of your cravings can make your body much less mysterious.

Sometimes, you'll be suffering from more than one nutrient imbalance that's causing a craving, and that can feel confusing. I want you to remember that your body already knows what it wants or needs; you just need to uncover what that thing is. When you read through the different possibilities, pause to feel what resonates the most with you. Start with that thing, and if it doesn't feel right when you're facing your craving, reread the section to find another possibility that resonates. Eventually, your body will open up to the right one, and poof! You know what your body is saying to you.

Sweet Foods

In general, I've found that people are either sweet or salt cravers, and the type of craving is kinda wired into each person. If the type of craving changes, like you've been a sweet craver and you start craving salty foods or vice versa, then you're experiencing a significant change that you need to pay attention to.

I'm a sweet craver who becomes a salt craver when the stress in my life becomes overwhelming, or I'm on the verge of burning out. (See Chapter 10 for information on burnout.) I've learned to identify my salt cravings as a red flag that I need to find some balance (while I also give my body what it needs by enjoying more sea salt).

Also, I don't consider my sweet cravings a "weakness," like many people feel their sweet cravings are. My body uses sweet foods for a specific purpose, and yours does, too.

I've found that many sweet cravers experience symptoms of low mood when they're stressed or overwhelmed, and they struggle terribly on a low-carb diet. The human body needs carbohydrates and starches for many reasons, and sweet cravers tend to have bodies that are particularly carb-friendly (healthy carb–friendly). Because sweets and carbs are currently out of fashion, having a carb-friendly body can be a big struggle in this protein-is-king world.

Sweet cravings can comfort us when we're feeling blue, and it's not only because of the feel-good loveliness of a sweet food melting on your tongue. There's a physiological reason for the comfort, too.

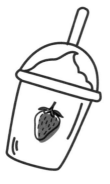

Your body uses protein, specifically the amino acid tryptophan, to make serotonin, the feel-good neurotransmitter. After a protein-heavy meal, your body is flooded with many different types of amino acids, and the lowly tryptophan, which is the least abundant amino acid, gets lost in the mix. However, after a starchy or sweet meal, insulin triggers all of the other amino acids to get pushed into your muscles, leaving tryptophan alone in your bloodstream, ready to be converted into serotonin. You literally get a mood boost when you eat sweets.

Your body digests refined sugary foods significantly faster than a starchy vegetable (like sweet potatoes). Although the boost in serotonin and the comforting effect are the same, the sugary food creates a spike in insulin, and then you feel a big crash, which leads to a craving for additional sweet foods. If you enjoy a high-fiber starchy vegetable instead of a handful of candy, you get a steady hit of serotonin without the crash. As I explain in Part 1, carbs/starches/sweet foods aren't created equally.

Aside from the mood-enhancer connection, there are a few other common sweet-craving connections to keep in mind. If you crave something sweet after meals, it could mean that your meal wasn't quite in balance for you. As I mentioned earlier, high-protein diets can be troublesome for sweet cravers, and a high-protein meal can trigger big-time sweet cravings as your body tries to rebalance that meal.

Sometimes your sweet cravings are due to a lack of sweetness and joy in your life. Your body is looking for a source of feel-goodness wherever it can find it, and eating sweet foods can feel so darn good. Consider whether your sweet craving might be linked to a deficit that can't be solved by food alone.

Not getting enough sleep is a common twenty-first-century deficiency that will make your body more insulin resistant and want sweet foods all day long. Research has found that people who don't sleep well are much more prone to being diagnosed with insulin resistance and type 2 diabetes. If you struggle with sleep, be extra wary of your sugar cravings and keep in mind that starchy veggies also curb your cravings but are much easier on your body.

WHAT TO DO

The most important thing I want you to remember when it comes to sugar cravings is that your body likes sweets and starchy carbs, and that's A-OK! You were probably born this way.

Don't let the mainstream diet-selling-machine scare you away from starchy food, like grains, potatoes, and other root veggies. They're out of style right now, but eventually, food styles will change, and carbs will be given a golden halo once again. In the meantime, enjoy whole-food carbs and starches, like potatoes (yes, they're good for you), sweet potatoes, root veggies, whole grains, and beans. And enjoy some fruit! Fruit is naturally sweet, delicious, and full of nutrients. Add them to your diet throughout the day to see how you feel. Your body will let you know what it needs.

DARK CHOCOLATE

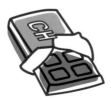

Dark chocolate is one of my top cravings and favorite foods all rolled into one. Cravings for dark chocolate can be connected to a magnesium deficiency because chocolate is really high in magnesium. (The body is just plain brilliant.) Although this connection between chocolate cravings and magnesium hasn't been proven scientifically, I've rarely found a person with an intense dark chocolate craving who didn't also have other symptoms of low magnesium.

If you crave dark chocolate, you're not alone! Chocolate cravings are the most common craving in North America, with 40 percent of women listing this delicious food as a major craving. Chocolate cravings can become more intense during the last week of a woman's menstrual cycle, which is another possible sign that the body is calling for more magnesium.

Other symptoms of low magnesium are tight muscles, leg cramps, exhaustion, and feeling phlegmy (having a stuffy nose and wet cough, for example).

Your body needs a lot of magnesium when you're stressed, eating junk food, or working out a lot, so it makes sense that I see symptoms of low magnesium a lot because people are frequently in one or more of these situations.

WHAT TO DO

Enjoy a few squares of dark chocolate one or two times per day. Use a high-quality cocoa or raw cacao in recipes, such as for a delicious chia or avocado pudding. Think of dark chocolate as a form of medicine rather than a "treat" you shouldn't have (gimme a WOO!). Nuts, seeds, avocado, and beans are also high in magnesium, so grab some extra servings of these foods, too.

MILK CHOCOLATE

Milk chocolate cravings can be very similar to dark chocolate cravings (a craving for magnesium), but milk chocolate comes with an added sugar hit. I've found that many people who love, love, LOVE milk chocolate deal with some blood sugar fluctuations, so their bodies are usually looking for a mix of magnesium and extra sugar.

WHAT TO DO

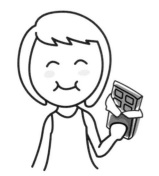

Consider a milk chocolate craving to be a magnesium craving–sugar craving tag team. Evaluate whether you have any other low-magnesium symptoms and add more magnesium-rich foods into your diet. (Check out the dark chocolate section for ideas.)

Also, consider swapping milk chocolate for a bar of dark chocolate that you really like. Dark chocolate usually contains much less sugar and other processed ingredients than milk chocolate, and it's usually satisfying after only a few squares (emphasis on *usually*). According to my clients (and my personal experience), the main issue with switching is the bitterness of dark chocolate. Some dark chocolate is very bitter, but many brands have a creamy sweetness. Look for dark chocolate bars that are about 70 percent cocoa—that's the sweet spot where health benefits and taste meet—and try a few to find one that you like.

CANDY

From my experience, candy cravings aren't your average sugar cravings; they always come alongside body pain. I can't think of a single example of someone I've worked with who had strong candy cravings but wasn't dealing with chronic body pain. So far, it's 100 percent.

Many years ago, I worked with a client who was a strong example of this connection. Jamie (a pseudonym) was dealing with severe digestive issues—so severe that Jamie was affected by the issues every day and had even made job decisions based on how close the bathroom was to their desk. These digestive issues had limited Jamie's diet to just a few foods—maybe five or six different things.

At some point in our conversation, Jamie asked if I minded if they stood up because they had a lot of back pain and sitting was becoming uncomfortable. As Jamie stood, I made an off-hand comment that they were the first person I had seen with chronic body pain who didn't have any candy cravings. That's when Jamie looked at me with a look of secrecy and whispered, "Well, I haven't told you about the jelly beans."

That's how strong the pain–candy craving connection can be; even for someone who had removed everything pleasurable from their diet to try to calm a loud and impatient gut, they still couldn't resist candy.

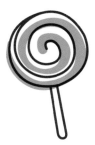

I've been doing a bit of an experiment with my clients for the last seven or eight years regarding this connection. (Don't worry; they're all in on the experiment.) I wanted to see which comes first: Does pain trigger sugar cravings? Or does sugar trigger pain?

I've talked to or heard from a few hundred people. So far, in about 95 percent of cases, it goes both ways. Pain triggers sugar cravings and refined sugar triggers pain. The good news is that you can break the cycle by pulling refined sugar out of your diet.

After a person has gone four to five days without any refined sugar, I've seen the average pain level go from an eight out of ten to a two or three. Many people have even reduced or eliminated their pain medications. It only takes four or five days to notice a difference, so it's a fast reward for the effort.

We know that sugar can trigger inflammation, and I'm sure that the candy must provide a nice serotonin boost, which helps relieve the pain for a few moments. Unfortunately, that fast hit of serotonin comes at a price—more pain in the future.

WHAT TO DO

If you want to try eliminating refined sugar to see if it has an effect on your pain level, remember one important point: Sweet foods aren't bad for you. It's only refined sugar (white sugar, cane sugar, high fructose corn syrup) that may be the problem. Throughout this experiment, give yourself sweet-tasting foods to help curb your cravings. Foods like fruit, unpasteurized honey, real maple syrup, dates, and sweet veggies (sweet potatoes, carrots, beets) can help curb your cravings for refined sugar.

Remove any foods that contain refined sugars. On food labels, you'll see them listed as sugar, glucose, fructose, sucrose (anything that ends with -ose), high fructose corn syrup, malt, syrups of any kind (except maple syrup), molasses, and maltodextrin. Look for them in all traditionally sweet foods (cookies, yogurt, and so on), but also look for them in foods you might not expect to have added sugar, such as bread, tomato sauce, granola, canned soup, and salad dressing.

Remove all refined sugar for five days to see how you feel. You have to commit 100 percent for this test to work, so be diligent. After five days, reintroduce your favorite sweet food to see if there's a change in your pain. If there is and you'd like to keep refined sugar out of your diet, slowly find alternatives for the foods you removed during your experiment. You don't have to make this happen overnight; just use the memory of how it felt to have less pain as your driver to keep going.

DEMANDING SUGAR CRAVINGS

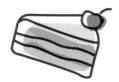

When you crave sweet foods, is that craving intense? Do you need to have your sugar fix NOW? Do you feel less patient or more frustrated until you get to enjoy some sweet, sweet goodness? If so, this isn't hunger or your average sweet craving; your cravings may happen in moments of lower blood sugar.

Your blood sugar goes up and down throughout the day with your meals, which is totally normal. It goes up a bit after you eat and then down a few hours later, which triggers hunger.

Real hunger feels like an empty feeling in your stomach, a slight dip in energy, and a feeling like, "I could eat something in the next hour or two." It's not demanding, and it doesn't affect your mood.

If your blood sugar goes up a bit too much after a meal, then it can dip too low afterward, triggering a very demanding craving for sweets—anything your body thinks you'll go out and get. It could be a favorite food (like chocolate), or it could be a convenient one (something handy). Your body will tempt you until you satisfy this craving.

WHAT TO DO

In the moment of a crash, try to stay as present as possible and only eat a small amount of food. Wait fifteen minutes before you eat anything else. You might feel like it's the longest fifteen minutes ever, and your body may keep tempting you to eat more and more food. If you give your body time to digest, though, you'll probably find your craving is satisfied.

I used to feel like this ALL. THE. TIME. It's so freeing to get off of the daily blood sugar roller coaster. So very freeing.

STEPPING OFF OF THE BLOOD SUGAR ROLLER COASTER

Dealing with a blood sugar crash at the moment is important, but the long-term solution is to keep your blood sugar balanced each day. With a few small tweaks, you can lessen or even eliminate those frustrating blood sugar crashes.

To get off the blood sugar roller coaster, focus on breakfast. Enjoying a good breakfast is the first important step to balancing your blood sugar. You'll just need to do some experimenting to find out what works best for you.

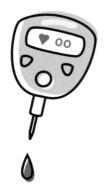

First, try to reduce how many super sugary foods you eat with breakfast, such as cereal, sweetened granola, sweetened nut butter, and sugar in your morning coffee or tea. Then add some protein, some healthy fat, and/or extra fiber to your breakfast. You can try eating a higher fat yogurt (look for one that has about 5 percent milk fat), eggs, avocado, or steel cut oats.

Try a few different breakfast options until you find one that you like *and* that keeps you feeling full and satisfied for at least four hours. If that doesn't solve all of your demanding sugar cravings, check out the section later in this chapter about afternoon cravings.

Salty Foods

▮ I have great news for all of the salt cravers out there! Salt cravings are cravings for...salt!

Salt has been vilified for decades, and a low-sodium diet has been promoted with very little proof that it's heart-healthy. This unsubstantiated nutritional advice has caused many salt cravers to deny their cravings for decades. That denial can lead to lots of cravings for processed salty foods, like pretzels, chips, and even pork rinds. Let's bring some healthy salt back into your diet!

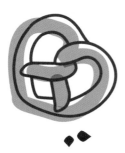

The words *salt* and *sodium* tend to be used interchangeably, but there's difference. Salt is a source of sodium chloride, but it isn't the only dietary source of sodium. Baking soda (sodium bicarbonate) is also a source of sodium (it's right there in the name), and most whole foods have naturally occurring sodium.

Please remember: *Humans need sodium!* The low-salt rhetoric has been so pervasive that people tend to forget this detail. Every single cell in your body depends on a balance of sodium and potassium, and the balance is so essential that your body will do whatever it takes to maintain it, including triggering a craving for salty food! You also need chloride, which is vital for many bodily functions, including making stomach acid and balancing fluid in your body. Sodium is an important electrolyte. You need salt!

Some people crave lots and lots of salt, and, in my experience, those people also tend to have low blood pressure. Salt helps you absorb water in your intestines, and it can help increase your blood volume. This is where the salt-equals-high-blood-pressure connection comes from, but there has been little research that has found that salt *causes* high blood pressure, other than observations of a temporary boost immediately after a person has consumed some salty food.

As in every other situation, your body is brilliant, and it's asking for what it needs. There's one thing you need to keep an eye on, though; you need to look at the quality of salt in your diet.

There is a time to reduce sodium in your diet. A small group of people are sensitive to sodium, and for those people, sodium can raise blood pressure too high. Always, always, always follow your doctor's advice. If your doctor has told you to follow a reduced-sodium diet, follow that advice until you've had a chance to discuss this new research with them.

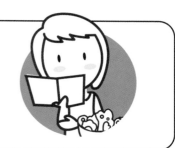

TABLE SALT VERSUS SEA SALT AND HIMALAYAN SALT

Sea salt is what it sounds like: the salt residue left behind by evaporated seawater. Sea salt naturally contains sodium chloride in a digestible form that's easy for your body to break apart and use. It also contains many trace minerals; the specific balance of minerals in sea salt depends on which sea the salt came from.

Himalayan or pink salt comes from the Kherwra Salt Mine. It's one of the largest salt mines in the world and is believed to come from an ancient body of water. Like sea salt, it's a natural salt that contains many trace minerals; some trace amounts of iron in the salt are responsible for its pink color.

Table salt, on the other hand, is highly refined to remove all of the impurities and trace minerals. It's pretty much pure sodium chloride with a bit of added iodine. Your body has a harder time breaking apart and digesting the sodium chloride, and the other beneficial minerals have been stripped from the salt during refining. Because table salt is hard to digest, your body may not get the benefit it's looking for, so your craving won't be satisfied.

Many people are concerned that switching to sea salt may create an iodine deficiency, but that's not necessarily true. The amount of iodine in salt is only a fraction of what you need each day, and it's not the best form of iodine. In the 1920s, manufacturers started adding the iodine to prevent goiter because options for getting sufficient iodine were limited. Now, much better sources of dietary iodine are available, such as wild fish, many vegetables, and seaweed.

WHAT TO DO

If you crave salt, enjoy it! (Unless your doctor has told you otherwise.)

If you eat a fairly healthy diet right now, you can use your taste buds as a guide. If your diet has a lot of processed foods and you currently eat fast food meals frequently, your taste buds might be a bit skewed. To transition, use some good quality sea salt, but not quite as much as you like, until your taste buds reset. A good sign that your taste buds have reset is when you start to miss vegetables after you've had a few less-than-healthy meals.

Many salt cravers also benefit from adding a pinch of sea salt to their water. This is especially important for people who tend toward low blood pressure. Once again, use your taste buds as a guide. When you need it, salted water will taste surprisingly refreshing rather than salty. If your salted water starts to taste unpleasantly salty, dump it out and pour a fresh glass of unsalted water.

POTATO CHIPS

Potato chip cravings can be connected to a few different body signals. You can be experiencing a salt craving, a carb craving, a calorie craving (because you haven't eaten enough in a day), a fat craving, or crunchy food craving.

Humans love a good crunch, so much so that food manufacturers spend a lot of time and money developing "the perfect crunch," which is why mainstream potato chips have a different crunch compared to small-batch kettle chips. Researchers have been looking at why people love noisy foods so much, and the current theory is that crunchy food exhibits freshness and crispness. Researchers have found that the louder the crunch of the food, the more people munch.

Potato chips can be comforting in many ways, so it's not always possible to nail down exactly what your body is asking for, but I have a few tricks for you.

WHAT TO DO

When you're craving some potato chips, you need to stay aware of the crunch-factor and the fact that chips are easy to overeat. Always eat a small portion out of a bowl of your own. Don't eat out of the bag, and don't share your bowl; doing those things will cause you to eat more. Enjoy every single bite and get more chips if you really need some. Deprivation isn't necessary, but you want to stay present inside this craving.

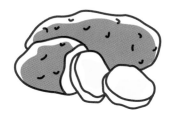

There are other ways to address a chip craving without actually eating chips. Roast a bunch of root veggies (like potatoes, sweet potatoes, carrots, beets, and so on) in olive oil or butter and lots of salt to solve a carb craving, fat craving, calorie craving, and salt craving; just know that the veggies won't be crunchy. I find this works most of the time, but not every time.

Strongly Flavored Snack/Junk Foods

According to food scientist Mark Schatzker in his book, *The Dorito Effect*, humans' taste buds have evolved to connect intense flavors with foods that are high in nutrients. When an apple, tomato, or pear is very flavorful, then it's also fully ripe and full of nutrients.

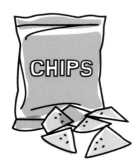

Today, the flavor of fruits and vegetables is diluted. For example, the taste of a freshly picked tomato from my garden bursts with flavor, but a tomato from the grocery store tastes milder. Food growers have traded more flavorful produce for larger and more pest-resistant produce varieties, because, frankly, uniformity and size make them more money. The exception to this trend is most farmer's markets, where unique heritage varieties are still king.

Now, the most flavorful foods on store shelves are usually highly processed junk foods, which explode with flavor on the tongue, but these foods are low in nutrients, so you're driven to eat more and more. Your body looks for the real nutrients in the nacho cheese flavoring of the chips as you crunch away on them, but those nutrients simply don't exist.

WHAT TO DO

If you find strongly flavored junk food irresistible, try adding nutrient-dense food to your diet, like more fruit, cooked veggies, and freshly pressed juices. Hopefully, your body will learn which foods are full of nutrients, so your craving shifts to those things. In the meantime, try to keep the junk foods out of your house (because they're manufactured to be addictive) or keep your serving size small. Don't eat out of the bag; instead, put some in a bowl and savor every bite.

Also, use the flavor you like as a guide to the foods to add to your diet. Do you love orange pop? Add more juicy navel oranges to your diet. Are nacho-flavored tortilla chips your weakness? Add more veggies like tomatoes and onions, high-quality cheese, and sea salt to your diet. Your taste buds and body need some time to get used to these blander foods, so be patient. Once your body shifts, the cravings will become less and less powerful.

Time of the Day Cravings

"Should I eat three meals and three snacks a day? Or just one meal? How important is the timing of meals?"

People ask me these questions a lot. Like, All. The. Time. Every nutrition expert seems to have an opinion on the subject of meal and snack frequency, and the conflicting information has become very confusing. Here's the truth as I see it: There's no one perfect answer. Everyone has unique needs for meal timing, but there are a few guidelines that work for most of us to help minimize cravings that crop up at particular times of the day.

Your body doesn't like to go very long periods without nourishment during the day because a lack of food puts stress on your system. If you wait more than five or six hours to eat between meals, your body needs to use cortisol, a stress hormone, to bring your blood sugar up. This system works well in the short term because it keeps your brain and body moving. Unfortunately, it uses up this precious stress hormone, which can trigger weight gain around your waist, and it can be a factor in burnout or adrenal fatigue, which I discuss in Chapter 10.

One popular recommendation is to eat three meals and three snacks every day to make sure your blood sugar never drops. But it's *exhausting* to prepare so many meals and snacks, and that system is hard to continue in the long term. Plus, you have to eat every two or three hours, and your digestive system never gets a break. Digesting all day long can zap energy and cause some digestive disturbances. If your blood sugar goes up and down all day, this three-meals-and-three-snacks system can be useful at first to balance blood sugar, but don't expect to continue it forever.

I recommend eating every four to five hours. Eat breakfast or something by 10:00 a.m. If eating breakfast makes you feel queasy, just have a snack mid-morning. Eat lunch by 1:00 p.m. and dinner by 7:00 p.m. That window of time between lunch and dinner is big (about six hours), so an afternoon snack can be handy around 4:00 p.m. This schedule gives enough space between meals to feel hungry but not so much that your body has to give you a zap of cortisol to bring your blood sugar up.

Some people feel best having only two meals a day, and that's okay, too. The key is balance. Be sure to eat enough food to stay fueled all day and that you eat frequently enough that all the day's food isn't crammed into one meal. Your digestive system doesn't like that very much.

Once you've found your prime mealtime schedule, you should notice that your energy stays steady all day, your mind is clear, and you have the energy to prepare each meal. But, if you find that your craving monster tends to visit you in the afternoon or in the evening, then you could be dealing with time of the day cravings.

AFTERNOON CRAVINGS

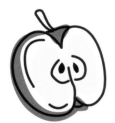

Afternoon cravings can be very demanding because of a one-two punch of hormones that happens in the afternoon. Cortisol, your energy hormone, is making its natural decline through the afternoon so you can sleep at night, and your blood sugar is also on its way down because you ate lunch so many hours earlier.

When you're tired and hungry when you drive home from work, you're probably tempted to stop off at a fast-food joint because it would be an easy solution. (Of course, major road-ways are lined with drive-through restaurants for this exact reason.) Or, if you make it home still hungry, your body may scream for a nice, relaxing (and blood-sugar-balancing) glass of wine. Your brain also reminds you of all of the delicious food in your cupboards, making it hard to stop a snacking session.

Lunch and dinner can be seven hours or more apart, so it's no wonder you want to dive headfirst into your cupboards after a long day at work. Everyone needs an afternoon snack, and this simple addition to your meal schedule can make cooking dinner much easier. It's an effective and easy change to make.

Always have a snack *before* you crash, around 3:30 or 4:00 p.m., and make it an energy-boosting snack to balance out the dip in blood sugar and cortisol. What's best? For most people, it's a piece of fruit, which is easy to grab and enjoy. Afternoon is also a good time of the day for a few squares of dark chocolate or a healthy homemade sweet treat.

EVENING CRAVINGS

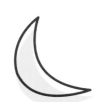

Oh, boy. There's certainly a lot of worry and judgment around evening cravings!

Evening is the time of the day when your willpower is low, and your body takes advantage of this moment to balance out any imbalances from earlier in the day. This is also a typical time for emotional cravings, and frequently evening cravings feel very emotional because usually you're not hungry (because you've recently had dinner).

Although emotional cravings are real, I've noticed that evening cravings are more often due to a body imbalance. When you rebalance, you can see more clearly which cravings are emotional and which are body cravings. So, at first, stay curious to determine the source of your evening cravings. I've tackled physical cravings throughout this chapter. If you realize that your cravings are emotional, seek out a professional who's trained to help you work through the emotions that trigger your craving.

When it comes to physical cravings, your body takes over in the evening to get what it wants or needs. When you sit down and relax, your body perks up and starts to send you cravings that were a lot easier to ignore earlier in the day when your mind was occupied on other things.

WHAT TO DO

In most cases, evening cravings are simple. They're a sign that you didn't eat enough during the day. Did you skip lunch? Are you reducing your food intake purposely? Did you eat enough starchy food for your body?

Replace the foods you're craving with healthier versions of those foods. How are your cravings when you eat more for breakfast? Or when you add some starchy food to your lunch? Let your body guide you, and you'll see what it's trying to tell you.

Interpreting Cravings

Your body is giving you signals each day to help you find balance. Use this handy guide to quickly interpret your cravings in the moment so you can give your body exactly what it's looking for.

CRAVING	WHAT IT MEANS	ALTERNATIVES
DARK CHOCOLATE	Low magnesium	70 percent dark chocolate, cocoa/cacao, nuts, seeds, beans, and avocado
MILK CHOCOLATE	Low magnesium, craving for sweetness	A dark chocolate you enjoy, or a homemade treat made with cocoa
CANDY	Possibly a serotonin boost, craving for sweetness	Fruit (like dates) and foods sweetened with honey, maple syrup, or other unrefined sugars
SALT	More salt!	Higher quality sea salt or Himalayan salt
POTATO CHIPS	More salt, carbs, or calories	Roasted root veggies with oil and salt
STRONGLY FLAVORED SNACK FOODS (like nacho cheese–flavored chips)	More nutrient-dense food	More veggies
AFTERNOON CRAVINGS	Low blood sugar and/or high stress	A high-energy 4:00 p.m. snack, like a piece of fruit
EVENING CRAVINGS	Not enough food through the day or a sign of emotional eating	Enjoy a healthy snack, but look for a pattern in other meals and address it

Wrapping It All Up

When it comes to your cravings, I want you to remember to stay curious. Instead of looking at cravings with frustration, look at them as information that needs to be uncovered or translated. Your cravings are a key piece of information for you to understand your body's language. Your body is guiding you to exactly which foods it wants so it can run optimally. It's yours to discover; just stay curious.

When you have a better understanding of your body's cravings, it's time to learn more about your digestive system and how to interpret its signs and signals. Your digestive system plays a key role in your overall health and will speak to you in its own language of symptoms whenever it needs a bit of support.

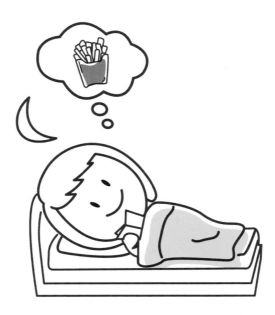

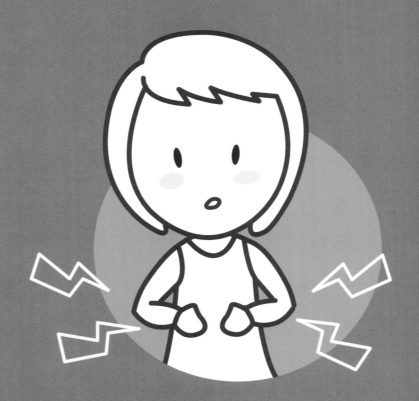

WHAT IS YOUR DIGESTIVE SYSTEM TELLING YOU?

"You are what you eat" has become a bit of a cliché, but the saying has a lot of truth to it. It needs one small tweak, though. I prefer the saying, "You are what you eat, digest, and assimilate."

Assimilate is the key part of that statement because your body can only use nutrients when they've been fully taken into your body. You can eat a beautiful and balanced diet, but if you're not properly assimilating your nutrients, then you might be dealing with deficiencies.

When your digestive system is happy, your whole body is happy! Better digestion gives you more energy, reduces inflammation, and reduces or eliminates all of your indigestion symptoms. It may even speed up your metabolism!

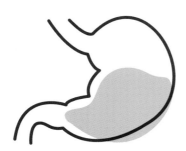

Your Microbiome Is Your Best Ally in Your Health

Some researchers estimate that half of the cells in your body are not human; they're bacteria. That bacteria community plays a huge role in your health. Most of the bacteria live in your digestive system; it's called the *microbiota* or *microbiome.*

Over the last few years, there's been a ton of research on the microbiome, but there are still a lot of unanswered questions. Studying this inner ecosystem is difficult because there are so many factors influencing it. There are about 1,000 different strains of bacteria working together as a community, so it's like studying the rain forest and trying to figure out which animal or plant species is the most important. As of writing this, scientists haven't found the strain or handful of strains of bacteria that create the "perfect" microbiome in everyone, and they probably never will.

Because your microbiome lives inside you, it's very determined that its home stays healthy and happy. When it's a strong, balanced community, the microbiome helps you digest your food, heals your gut walls, balances your immune system, adjusts your metabolism, and even affects how you think.

The Gut/Brain Connection

Your microbiome is surrounded by a sea of neurons or nerve cells. More neurons live around your gut than in your spine. This enteric nervous system (ENS), which you can refer to as a "second brain," is so vast and complex that it makes most of your neurotransmitters (your brain's chemical messengers), including 90 percent of your serotonin and 50 percent of your dopamine. Research is finding that gut bacteria play a role in keeping your body's neurotransmitters in balance and maintaining good mental health. In your gut, these neurotransmitters help you digest your food.

It's hard to imagine that your gut health would affect your brain, but research has found that having irritable bowel syndrome (IBS) is connected with a greater chance of having a psychiatric disorder. As of this writing, anxiety and diarrhea are both thought to be triggered by an abundance of neurotransmitters, and depression and constipation are thought to be due to an absence of neurotransmitters.

What I find to be the coolest area of research is how your gut bacteria may change your personality. When timid mice were inoculated with gut bacteria from adventurous mice, they quickly became adventurous, too. And the adventurous mice became timid as soon as they were given gut bacteria from the timid mice. A study from The Ohio State University looked at stool samples from toddlers and found those with the most diverse inner ecosystem had the most positive behavioral attributes. They were more likely to be cooperative and share their toys.

This study also found a possible correlation between diverse gut bacteria and extroversion in the boys in the group. I come from a family of introverts, and I identify on the introverted side of the scale, and it made me wonder whether my introversion is something in my genes or that was a trait passed on to me through my mom's gut bacteria?

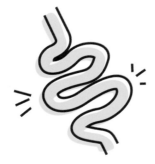

The Gut/Immune Connection

The bacteria in your gut are technically foreign invaders, so shouldn't the immune system kill them off? That's its job—to find foreign cells, like suspicious bacteria, and eliminate them. In the case of these foreign invaders, your microbiome has developed not only a symbiotic relationship with your immune system but it's taken charge.

Early mammals had an organized microbiome long before the immune system developed. As the early mammalian bodies developed a primitive immune system, the microbiome took the reins to keep its home safe and sound. To make sure that the bacteria weren't kicked to the curb by the immune system, the microbiome took over the job of deciding when the immune system should attack. It's your immune system's modulator; your microbiome tells your immune system when to attack and when to stand down. Think about that for a moment: Cells that aren't human but dwell in your body are what decide how your immune system functions.

Scientists can't really determine what a human's life would be like without a microbiome because there's no way to study it in humans. Forcing a person to live without a functioning microbiome would be cruel, but (sadly) researchers can perform animal studies to see what happens. Germ-free mice have been found to have a blunted immune system, and they aren't able to respond appropriately to an invader.

In humans, researchers are beginning to connect an imbalance in the microbiome with many inflammatory diseases and autoimmune conditions. Currently, there's a proposed connection between the clean lifestyle found in North America and the rising number of kids diagnosed with type 1 diabetes (which is an autoimmune disease). A six-fold increase in this condition was found in kids who had clean water to drink and lived in homes with proper sanitation compared to those who had many strains of bacteria in their drinking water and a childhood rife with many intestinal infections. Also, early research is connecting a change in gut bacteria with age-related chronic inflammation.

I believe we're going to see more and more research into this area over the next few decades, and we may soon see probiotics, fermented foods, and other dietary measures used as the mainstream treatment for many autoimmune and inflammatory conditions that are currently very hard to treat. We still have a long way to go to uncover the power of the gut/immune connection.

Your Microbiome Affects the Energy You Extract from Food

The discovery of antibiotics has played a major role in human health. Antibiotics were a breakthrough for treating bacteria-based diseases and formerly deadly childhood diseases, such as meningitis and strep throat, that are easily cured with antibiotics. However, it's now become apparent that we've been overusing them. Antibiotic-resistant bugs are creeping in and are quickly becoming deadly. Often, people blame doctors for over-prescribing antibiotics, but agriculture is where the majority of the antibiotics are used in North America.

Beginning in the mid-1950s, conventional animal producers fed subtherapeutic doses of antibiotics to their animals daily, not to ward off infection but to fatten them up. Could the antibiotic residue found in these foods when we eat them be unintentionally doing the same thing to us?

Thankfully, this method of fattening up animals is changing. In 2017, the U.S. Food and Drug Administration banned the use of antibiotics in animals for growth. The antibiotic residue found in food has reduced by one-third since the change took effect.

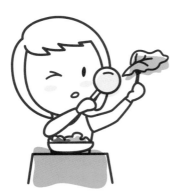

Dr. Martin Blaser, Director of NYU's Human Microbiome Project, proposes in his book *Missing Microbes* that a steady intake of prescription antibiotics, antibiotic residue, and anti-microbial compounds in the diet (like chlorine on salad greens) are the cause of weaker microbiomes, and this may be affecting metabolism (as well as the immune system and other body systems). In his research, mice given antibiotics early in life gain weight much faster than those with an intact microbiome. The question is, if this affects mice, does it affect humans as well?

Your Gut Bacteria Balance Is in Your Hands

Scientists may never find the "perfect" microbiome balance, just like they may never find the balance of trees and wildlife that makes up the perfect forest. My microbiome is as unique as a fingerprint and is balanced to suit my diet, my climate, and my interaction with other lovely humans. That's the goal: to make your microbiome perfect for *you.*

You have a lot of control over your microbiome. Sometimes you indeed need antibiotics to deal with an infection, and that feels a bit out of your control, but there's a lot you can do every day to help balance your inner ecosystem.

Most importantly, your bacteria eat whatever you eat, and your diet plays a huge role in determining both the strains of bacteria that take up residence in and the diversity of your microbiome. They munch mostly on undigested fiber, and your good bacteria especially love plant-based fiber from veggies, fruits, nuts, seeds, beans, and grains. The American Gut Project has found that diets with the highest diversity of plant-based fiber feed the most diverse microbiomes.

Fermented foods, like sauerkraut, whole milk yogurt, and kefir, fertilize your gut beautifully. These foods are full of good bacteria but not of the type of bacteria that takes up residence. Bacteria from these foods are usually transient, but that's not a bad thing! As the bacteria move through your gut, they leave in their wake an amazing environment for a robust and diverse ecosystem. Research has found that regularly eating fermented foods is linked to a diverse microbiome.

Many people unknowingly stress their microbiomes by eating a low-fiber diet or inadvertently eating foods with antibiotic residue. Without a steady supply of fiber, the good bacteria in your colon can die off, and other refined-food-lovin' but less-than-stellar strains can take their place.

It doesn't take long to make real changes in your microbiome! Research has found that within four days of a dietary shift, a person's gut bacteria has noticeably changed. Wherever your microbiome is today, it can be well on its way to better balance in just one short week.

Evaluating Your Digestion

Everyone feels some digestive symptoms from time to time. Pay attention to any symptoms you feel regularly and notice anytime they're getting stronger. By recognizing the symptoms when they're happening, you're making your gut happier. Most of the time, it just wants to be heard.

The following are some common symptoms of digestive issues:

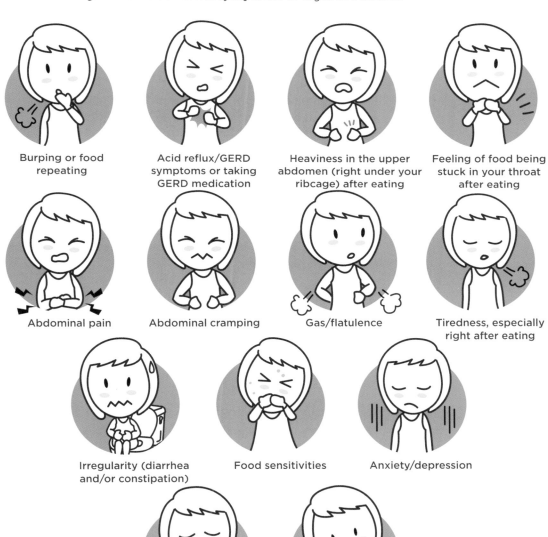

Burping or food repeating

Acid reflux/GERD symptoms or taking GERD medication

Heaviness in the upper abdomen (right under your ribcage) after eating

Feeling of food being stuck in your throat after eating

Abdominal pain

Abdominal cramping

Gas/flatulence

Tiredness, especially right after eating

Irregularity (diarrhea and/or constipation)

Food sensitivities

Anxiety/depression

Chronic inflammation

Slow metabolism

Each digestive organ has its own language, and by understanding which organ is "talking," you can more easily understand what your body is trying to say. Sometimes it can be easier to hear your colon (irregularity) than your stomach, but if your stomach is unhappy, it can cause problems all through your digestive system. Tune in and listen to everything your body would like to tell you.

STOMACH

The stomach is a very acidic place, and it completes an important step in digestion. This acid finishes the job that your teeth started when they broke down (or maybe didn't break down, if you didn't chew well) big chunks of food. The acid and enzymes also work on any protein in your meal to break it down and bind it with minerals so they can be absorbed in your small intestine.

Your whole digestive system reacts to stress, but this effect is particularly strong in your stomach.

Your brain primarily controls your stomach, whereas your ENS (that "second brain" in your gut) controls the rest of your digestive system. When your brain perceives stress, your stomach also gets the message.

For some people, stress can shut down the stomach's digestive process, which results in feelings of heaviness, overfullness, food reflux, or bloating in the upper abdomen. For others, it triggers an overproduction of stomach acid, which can cause burning, pain, and all of the unpleasantness of severe acid reflux.

Your digestive habits, or how you eat, can help relieve stomach symptoms. Good habits can take some practice to adopt, but your stomach will thank you. I explain good digestive habits in the "Three Steps to a Gut Reset" section later in this chapter.

SMALL INTESTINE

After your food leaves your stomach, it heads to the small intestine, which is where most of your food gets fully broken down and absorbed into your body. The small intestine is an important place; it's the spot for assimilation.

To make sure your food has space to be digested and absorbed, your small intestine has a *giant* surface area. If your small intestine were stretched out flat, it would be about the size of a small tennis court!

There's a small but important ecosystem of bacteria living here. It's only one cell layer thick, but it provides enormous protection for the epithelial layer in your small intestine (which, amazingly, is also only one cell layer thick). The epithelial layer is the top layer of your intestinal wall, where the digested food and nutrients in your digestive system move into your body and bloodstream.

This bacteria community also assists by producing extra enzymes to help you digest your food (like lactase to digest dairy). Your bacteria help to heal your gut lining, and they communicate with your immune system to alert it if there's a rogue invader, like a virus, trying to get through.

If you have undigested sugars in your small intestine, then you might feed bad bacteria and yeast (like candida). If this is happening, you also (usually) feel a lot of gas and bloating. This gas might blow up your intestine like a balloon and often is very visible (it can make you look pregnant).

If you have undigested protein in your small intestine and it "leaks" through a damaged spot in your epithelial layer, your immune system can be triggered. This issue is sometimes called a "leaky gut." This immune reaction can trigger seasonal allergy symptoms, inflammation, and possibly autoimmune issues.

Undigested fat in the small intestine doesn't cause too much trouble. It doesn't trigger bloating or inflammation; it just slides on through. However, it can overlubricate your gut, which can trigger a fast and fatty bowel movement. If this happens to you, add some digestive bitters such as dandelion greens and ginger, to your routine to support your gall bladder and fat digestion.

YOUR COLON AND IRREGULARITY

The best way to assess your digestive process is by paying attention to what goes into your digestive system (what you eat) and how it comes out (your poop).

Your gut and brain are also very connected, and anxiety and depression can trigger digestive symptoms as well. Generally speaking, anxiety and diarrhea are connected, and depression and constipation are connected. However, everyone's gut is unique, so don't worry if you're a constipated anxious person or vice versa.

Diarrhea

Diarrhea is a sign that your body is trying to get rid of something and/or you're feeling super anxious. Urgency (needing to go NOW!) is a big sign your body doesn't like something you've eaten lately. Although this is a *very* frustrating and debilitating symptom, it does balance out pretty quickly once you rebalance your gut bacteria and figure out your trigger food(s).

To start, keep a food diary and keep track of your symptoms. Does a pattern emerge? If you notice a pattern of certain food culprits or stress that seem to be triggering your symptoms, try removing them from your diet or altering your lifestyle as you continue to keep track of your symptoms. If your symptoms lessen or go away completely, then you'll know you found the culprit. Success!

Constipation

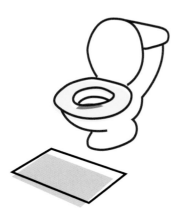

Constipation is a bit trickier to address than diarrhea, but balance is possible. A lack of fiber often takes the blame as the culprit, but if you're eating a fair number of veggies, then that's probably not your issue. Most people I work with are already eating enough fiber, and adding more just makes the problem worse.

From my experience, most constipation issues with healthy eaters (or healthy-ish eaters) stem from dehydration, not eating enough fat, or not having enough of the right bacteria. Rebalancing these elements usually works well.

Another little trick to help with constipation is to elevate your knees when you're on the toilet. Your body was meant to squat while eliminating, and it's believed that an important muscle—the puborectalis muscle—doesn't fully relax when you sit. This muscle contracts around your colon when you're standing to stop any feces from getting out. It relaxes fully when you squat, allowing for a much easier bowel movement. If you want to know more, check out the instructional videos by the company Squatty Potty on YouTube. If you'd like to try elevating your knees while you're on the toilet, any step stool works like a charm.

Multiple Issues

If you have symptoms in each part of your digestive system, you're not alone! If your stomach isn't working very well, it can trigger a cascade of symptoms all through your digestive system. Start at your stomach (or small intestine if that's the first spot where you experience symptoms) and work your way down. You'll be surprised to see colon symptoms disappear after your stomach is working better.

DIGESTIVE ORGAN	SYMPTOMS	SOLUTION
STOMACH	GERD/acid reflux, burping, nausea, heaviness under or just below your ribcage, regurgitation, feeling like food is stuck in your throat	Practice good digestive habits
SMALL INTESTINE	Gas, cramping, bloating, abdominal pain, food sensitivities, lactose intolerance, slow metabolism, chronic inflammation	Enjoy gut-bacteria-supportive foods, increase lactobacillus bacteria
COLON	Irregularity, cramping, pain, mental health issues	Enjoy gut bacteria-supportive foods, consider using a foot stool to elevate your knees when you're on the toilet, increase bifidobacteria

Three Steps to a Gut Reset

If you're experiencing issues somewhere in your digestive system, this gut reset is an effective way to address them, even if you only do it slowly, one part at a time. You don't need to follow the steps in order; just start wherever you feel most comfortable and add a new step when you're ready. Plus, you might find all you need is one step and voilà! Your gut is happy again! Your gut is pretty darn amazing.

DIGESTIVE HABITS AND A TRANSIT TIME TEST

Making the following changes is valuable, especially if you experience a lot of stomach symptoms. It's also surprisingly difficult to do, so be really kind to yourself.

Be as relaxed as possible while you're eating: You're either stressed *or* digesting. Take a moment, a deep breath, and sink into the meal you're about to have.

Chew, chew, chew—your stomach doesn't have teeth: Chewing your food well helps your stomach enormously. Large chunks of food are difficult to digest using only stomach acid and digestive juices. Always keep in mind that your stomach doesn't have any teeth. A little trick to make this easier is to put your fork down between bites because that action automatically slows you down.

No (or very little) liquids with meals: Drinking a lot while you eat dilutes your stomach acid and makes it much harder to digest your food. Plus, liquids overfill your stomach, which can trigger acid reflux/GERD symptoms. Drink no more than ½ cup of liquid with your meal, and wait at least an hour before drinking more.

If you notice that you're eating quickly, just put your fork down and try again. It takes a few weeks for these habits to come more easily. When you eat slowly and chew a meal thoroughly, notice how you feel. When you eat a meal in a rush or too quickly, take note of how you feel then, too. Being curious about how you feel can make this process easier.

Bonus Step, transit time test: Your digestion might be sluggish or too fast, and an easy way to know what's going on is by doing an easy transit time test to determine how long food takes to pass through your digestive system from your mouth to the toilet. Repeat this test every few months to keep an eye on your transit time.

- Eat about 1 cup of corn or beets and write down the time and day you ate the food.

- Watch for that food to appear in your stool and write down the day and time you see the last of the corn or beets.

Healthy transit time is eighteen to twenty-four hours (but it can be up to forty-eight hours if you've dealt with chronic constipation).

GUT BACTERIA-SUPPORTIVE FOODS

Keep your inner ecosystem/microbiome healthy and strong by feeding them their favorite foods, such as probiotics, plant-based fiber, and fermented foods. It doesn't take long to feel the difference!

A Good Probiotic Supplement

By "good," I mean one that works for you. You should feel a reduction in your digestive symptoms within one month (usually within a few weeks) of starting to take a probiotic supplement. If you don't, try a different one. I like multi-strain, human-strain probiotic supplements. If your symptoms seem to be related to your stomach or small intestine, look for a supplement with lots of *lactobacillus* bacteria. If your colon is your main concern, look for one that's full of bifidobacteria.

Plant-Based Fiber (aka Prebiotics)

You don't need to buy a fancy supplement to get prebiotic fiber. You just need to eat lots of veggies, fruit, whole grains, beans, and nuts and seeds. All of these foods are chock-full of prebiotic fiber, which is the food of choice for your gut bacteria. Ground flax and chia seeds are particularly gut-bacteria-friendly.

Fermented Foods

Fermented foods contain both good bacteria *and* prebiotic fiber. They also leave a wonderful environment for your gut bacteria in their wake. Just one serving per day is all you need!

Fermented foods like kefir, unpasteurized sauerkraut, fermented veggies, yogurt, kombucha, or tempeh are excellent sources of good bacteria and fiber. Find a fermented food you love and enjoy!

EXTRA GUT-HEALING FOODS

Some foods can help to soothe your gut and reduce the symptoms that you're feeling. You don't need to use all of them. Just find one or two that help with the symptoms you're feeling and make them a regular part of your diet.

Slippery Elm

This simple powder is like a soothing balm for your gut. It can heal any painful, irritated spots. It's also a great regulator for your colon and helps with both constipation and diarrhea. It's best for pain, cramping, and irregularity.

Take 1 teaspoon to 1 tablespoon in water, one to four times per day. Give the slippery elm one to three days to start working (although some people feel some relief almost immediately).

Aloe Vera Juice

Taking aloe vera juice internally is like putting aloe gel on a burn on your skin. It's cooling and soothing. It's excellent for a tender esophagus that's been damaged by acid reflux, and it's also helpful for healing leaky gut. It can be helpful after radiation as well. Take 2 to 4 ounces, two times per day.

> Ingesting aloe vera juice is not for anyone with latex or aloe allergies. If you're in that group, a great alternative is 5 grams per day of L-glutamine powder.

Gut-Healing Chia Pudding

Chia pudding is a delicious treat that also helps the gut—my favorite combination. When soaked, chia seeds produce a gel-like fiber, which feeds good bacteria and can regulate the gut.

Chia pudding works best for alleviating constipation or diarrhea. Just enjoy ½ to 1 cup each day! (For a homemade version, you can try the recipe at my website: lisakilgour.com/articles/2019/1/21/healing-chia-chocolate-pudding.)

Wrapping It All Up

Your gut speaks to you each day in myriad ways, and by learning its language, you can better understand any early signs of indigestion. By really optimizing your digestion, you'll absorb and assimilate more nutrients from the food you eat, while also supporting your inner ecosystem (your microbiome), which supports many organs and body systems. Supporting your digestive system is vital for a healthy and vibrant body.

All of this knowledge of your cravings and digestion is great, but what if you're so tired you're barely getting through your day? It's a very taxing time to be alive, and more and more people are finding that low energy or fatigue are daily problems. Coming up next, learn what your body is looking for when your energy dips and how to heal your inner energy system so you can feel like your old, superstar self again.

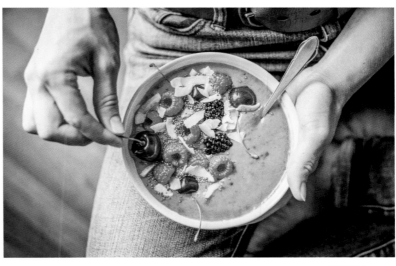

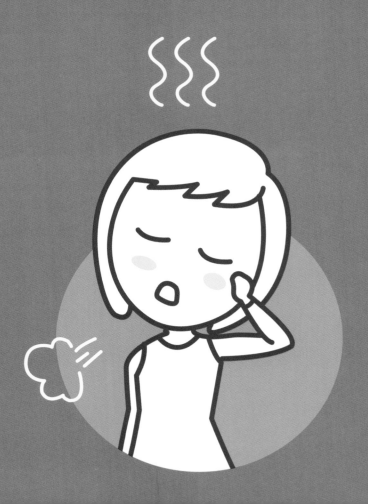

WHAT IS YOUR ENERGY LEVEL TELLING YOU?

How have you been feeling lately? Dig deep and really feel it for a second. Are you feeling fantastic? Do you jump out of bed every morning ready to tackle the day? Or have you been feeling less than amazing? Do you have a bad case of the blahs or the I-don't-wannas? Feeling downright tired? Dragging yourself through your day and just barely getting by?

If you're feeling fantastic—wonderful! Sadly, you're a rare exception in the world today. Most people report feeling either tired or totally exhausted. Chronic exhaustion is so common that it has become normal, and "busy" has become a frequent response to, "How are you doing?"

I know this feeling, too. As I mentioned in the Introduction, as a self-employed adrenaline junkie, I've burned myself out more than once. The first time I burned out, I lived in a fog that I accepted as normal. (Like it's "normal" to be so foggy that I'd forget what day of the week it was and where I was going.) I felt so foggy that retrieving any information from my brain was difficult. Frankly, I was lucky to remember my name during that time.

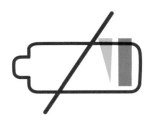

Recovering from my first experience with burnout was the beginning of my journey toward becoming a holistic nutritionist. It was my first time diving into the world of nutrition, and I was hooked, so much so that I eventually went back to school to formally study it. Well, I became a not-so-perfect holistic nutritionist because I burned out again while building my wellness business. This time, though, I caught myself in an earlier stage of burnout and healed much faster.

I feel it's important to be open and honest about my experience with adrenal fatigue and burnout. I feel we need to talk about all of our experiences because so many people are silently dealing with these problematic symptoms. In fact, the number of people who are dealing with full-blown adrenal exhaustion in my consulting practice has skyrocketed in the last few years. And the number of people I see who are feeling so exhausted they're close to being bedridden has *seriously* skyrocketed. Instead of seeing a few people in total burnout each year, I now see a few each month, which is about a tenfold increase.

Burnout

In 2019, the World Health Organization (WHO) listed burnout as an "occupational phenomenon" in its eleventh revision of the International Classification of Diseases (ICD). This designation was a big deal to me because a condition that so many people have been dealing with had finally been recognized by mainstream medicine. The condition's inclusion in the ICD made it real in the eyes of many medical professionals.

WHO has defined burnout as

...a syndrome conceptualized as resulting from chronic workplace stress that has not been successfully managed. It is characterized by three dimensions:

- *feelings of energy depletion or exhaustion;*

- *increased mental distance from one's job, or feelings of negativism or cynicism related to one's job; and*

- *reduced professional efficacy.*

Burn-out refers specifically to phenomena in the occupational context and should not be applied to describe experiences in other areas of life." (Definition courtesy of the World Health Organization)

Although calling burnout an occupational phenomenon isn't a diagnosis, I do think this is a huge step in the right direction when it comes to humans' health and lifestyles. Now workplaces must consider that their environment and culture affect the health and productivity of the company's workers. Despite what the WHO definition says, people don't feel burned out only because of workplace stress. What this definition misses is all of the other stress that people experience in life. For most of us, stress comes from a combination of a stressful work environment and busy lives at home. To me, this definition is missing the personal element, but it's a start.

CURRENT LIFESTYLES AND THE INEVITABILITY OF BURNOUT

Life is a lot busier today than it was even one generation ago. I was raised in the 1980s in a typical suburban middle-class family. My dad worked forty hours a week at his job, and my mom worked at home to take care of my big sister and me until I was almost ten. We weren't rich, but we had a comfortable house, a kitchen full of food, and even a few vacations. Of course, I don't know very much about my parents' actual financial situation, but in my eyes, it seemed like we easily survived off of my dad's salary.

Today, people often live a lot differently. Most families need two incomes to afford that same lifestyle I grew up with. And, the forty-hour workweek has become a rarity. Instead, it's become the norm to handle double or triple the workload of a generation ago. If you've survived an all-too-common corporate layoff, then you're also expected to be grateful to have that huge workload. People are often tied to their phones all evening and answer work emails right up until bedtime. Workers no longer think it's unusual to feel stress or anxiety whenever they're away from their phones for any length of time.

In other words, it's become so routine to feel absolutely and completely exhausted that those feelings are almost unnoticeable.

Sadly, the consensus tends to be that a person who has the completely reasonable feelings of burnout and exhaustion is weak or has something wrong with them. People internalize those judgments, and the result is that they might feel that they can't handle things as well as everyone else. I'm here to tell you a truth: The only "normal" thing to feel in this crazy go-go-go world is feeling burned out. If that's how you feel, you have nothing to be ashamed of. Most of your colleagues, friends, and coworkers feel the same way. If you assume everyone else is coping with the stress while you're not, please know that you're not alone.

I talk to people every day who feel shame in their exhaustion even though most people feel the same way. This collective feeling of exhaustion is a reasonable reaction to the idolization of "busy." This shame surrounding our collective exhaustion is a reaction to a time where rest, play, and joy are viewed as being "lazy," and we're all constantly being bombarded by everyone else's accomplishments and successes over social media.

Let me say it one more time: It's normal to feel exhausted. You've earned your exhaustion by being unbelievably capable. You've earned it by being an absolute *superstar*. If you're feeling exhausted, your body is telling you (as politely as it can) that it needs some replenishing. It needs some help.

THE MYTH OF HIGH ENERGY

Today there's a coffee shop on every corner and energy drinks in every gas station. It's no wonder people have a skewed sense of high energy. I've spent years in a super high-energy state myself. I'm sensitive to caffeine, but that didn't stop me from downing an energy booster first thing in the morning, black tea on my way to the office, and another energy booster before my workout. I'm a naturally high-energy, fast-talking person, and anyone who knows me would prefer I be less caffeinated when I'm in their presence. (I'm not joking; I've been asked not to drink coffee before coming to at least two different workplaces.)

So, why did I hype myself up with caffeine all the time? It's a simple reason: I fell victim to the high-energy myth like a lot of people do. I was under the belief that super high energy was a "normal" state. Man, I was so wrong.

I see this misconception in a lot of my clients—especially my clients who are in their twenties. I've seen people who have an overall healthy diet struggle to stop their energy drink habit, and many people have a caffeine intake well over 300 milligrams per day! (For reference, an 8-ounce mug of coffee is about 95 milligrams of caffeine.) I've also seen a significant number of twenty-somethings dealing with many symptoms of adrenal fatigue, which I talk about later in this chapter.

When I started working as a nutritionist, all of my clients with adrenal fatigue symptoms were in their fifties, so it was shocking when I started to see twenty-somethings burn out so quickly. But many younger people are working two or three jobs while dealing with school full time, so it's no wonder they're burning out.

People are living inside the myth that being super busy and super energetic equals being productive and successful. I believe that's not always the case, though. In my case, my productivity skyrocketed once I traded my caffeine habit for meditation, and I'd describe the way I felt as being more balanced than super energetic. Feeling calm and clear-headed is a more comfortable state, and I'm no longer riding on the high of caffeine and adrenaline all day. As a former lover of high-energy caffeine, I wouldn't trade this feeling of calm and balance for anything.

BURNOUT AND ADRENAL FATIGUE

Both adrenal fatigue and burnout are syndromes, not diseases, so there's no accurate blood test or scan that you can do to see how your body is handling stress. Instead, you might experience a range of symptoms that can get progressively worse until you make some changes.

Until the WHO declared burnout as a real condition, in the world of nutrition, we mostly talked about adrenal fatigue, which is a syndrome that has not been recognized whatsoever in mainstream medicine, even though the symptoms are real and very unpleasant.

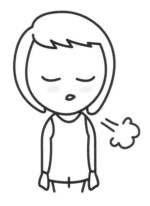

Burnout has been described as a feeling of exhaustion and mental distance from one's job. Adrenal fatigue shares these symptoms, and other physical symptoms usually manifest as well. Low blood pressure, anxiety, depression, salt and/or sugar cravings, muscle tension, and brain fog are typical symptoms of adrenal fatigue.

The adrenal glands are tiny triangle organs that live on top of your kidneys and manage your stress response. They kick in to provide adrenaline and cortisol anytime you're in a situation that calls for the fight-or-flight response. Cortisol affects you all day long by helping you wake up in the morning, increasing your blood pressure when you stand up, and playing a role in balancing your blood sugar.

When you're under chronic stress, your cortisol levels can be high all day, which leads to high blood pressure, high blood sugar, and a few extra pounds around your belly. Adrenal fatigue describes the moment when your adrenals can't keep up anymore, and your cortisol level dips. Many people feel symptoms of adrenal fatigue for years despite having cortisol levels still within the appropriate range, which is where the controversy lies.

A naturopath or functional medicine doctor can help diagnose adrenal fatigue. These practitioners use a variety of tools to make the diagnosis, including administering a cortisol spit or urine test, tracking blood pressure changes (postural hypotension when your blood pressure drops when you stand up), and running some blood work. Adrenal fatigue syndrome can present itself differently from person to person, so a holistic whole-body approach is needed to identify and treat it.

IDENTIFYING ADRENAL FATIGUE

The symptoms of adrenal fatigue are really varied and surprisingly common. Here's a list of the common symptoms that can be signs of adrenal fatigue. Take a look and see how your adrenals are doing:

- **Salt cravings:** Whether you're a long-time salt craver or a new one, any increase in your salt cravings can be a sign that your adrenals are getting tired or are overwhelmed. Your adrenals manage your blood pressure; they raise it when you're under stress and lower it when you're relaxed. Good-quality sea or Himalayan salt is a very medicinal food for your adrenals. Remember, salt cravings are truly a craving for salt!

- **Light-headedness:** This symptom tends to arrive later than salt cravings, and the light-headedness is related to the salt deficiency. As your adrenals get tired, they struggle to keep your blood pressure up, especially when you stand up suddenly, such as after tying your shoes. Light-headedness can be caused by many things, so please talk with your doctor about this before assuming you're suffering from adrenal fatigue.

- **Wired but tired:** Have you ever felt tired all day but then felt wide awake once you go to bed? If you're thinking, "Heck, yes!" then you're not alone. This is a common symptom of adrenal fatigue, and many women experience it during perimenopause. As your adrenals heal and your cortisol levels start to balance out, you *will* sleep again.

- **Extra jumpy/easily overwhelmed:** This is one of the first red flags that lets me know I need to cut back on caffeine and introduce some relaxation. I get jumpy when I drive, but other people might startle easily from loud noise, a sudden change in temperature (like going outside into the heat or cold), or just feeling like their "nerves are fried."

- **Big energy crash mid-afternoon:** It's common to feel a bit hungry or a little sleepy in the afternoon. This is a time where your cortisol levels are naturally on their way down so you can sleep at night, and your blood sugar drops after lunch. That combo can make it hard to concentrate in the late afternoon. But, if you feel T-I-R-E-D and/or hangry (so hungry it affects your mood), then you're receiving a sign that your adrenals might be getting tired. Until you're feeling better, try not to book any difficult or creative work or high-stress tasks for the late afternoon.

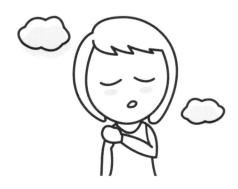

If you're experiencing any of these symptoms or feeling extra tired lately, and you're concerned you might be dealing with burnout or adrenal fatigue, it's a good idea to visit your general practitioner to rule out a few issues. These are conditions that can be easily diagnosed through a blood test, and they share a lot of symptoms with adrenal fatigue:

- **Low iron/anemia:** When your iron is low, your blood struggles to carry enough oxygen. This can lead to a deep sense of exhaustion, brain fog, and being easily winded. Check your hemoglobin and ferritin levels to see whether low iron is causing your symptoms.

- **Hypothyroid:** Your thyroid manages your metabolism, body temperature, and energy. When your thyroid is low, you can feel *tired*! Have your doctor take a look at your TSH, T3, and T4 levels to see how your thyroid is doing.

Fast Energy Boosters

If you're feeling totally exhausted and would rate your energy at a three or lower out of ten, you can try some fast energy boosters. Don't worry about making any major dietary changes right now; just add a few easy foods to your diet to feed your body some extra energy and nutrients.

These natural, nonstimulating energy boosters will bring your energy up enough so you can work through the long-term healing. The following suggestions are listed in order of effectiveness:

- **Sea salt (lots and lots of sea salt):** Salt isn't the villain you've been told it is. It's actually very healing, especially for your adrenal glands. Remember, though, that there's a world of difference between sea salt and table salt. Table salt is highly processed, and only sea salt (or Himalayan salt) is medicinal. Add it to your food to your taste (especially if you're craving salt). You also can try adding a pinch to your water, which is particularly helpful if you're feeling dizzy due to low blood pressure.

- **4:00 p.m. snack:** Everyone needs a 4:00 p.m. snack, but it's especially helpful if you're feeling exhausted. Lunch and dinner are way too far apart, and your cortisol and blood pressure are on their natural decline in the afternoon. Consequently, you're extra tired and foggy. When you can, grab a piece of fruit, dark chocolate, veggie juice, or a handful of nuts and eat it before you're feeling hangry.

- **Fresh veggie juices:** There's a time and a place for fresh-pressed veggie juices, and when you're exhausted is exactly the time and place. Juicing gives your body *tons* of nutrients without making it go through all of the work digesting the food. Head to a juice bar or borrow a juicer to see if this feels good to you. All fresh veggie juice combos are good for you, so find one that tastes delightful. More veggies, less fruit is best for your blood sugar.

- **Fruit, fruit, glorious fruit:** Fruit is *so* good for you when you're tired! It's chock-full of vitamins, it's super hydrating, and it has just enough sugar to give you a boost along with stabilizing fiber. It's an easy high-energy snack. Enjoy two to four pieces of fruit each day, especially if you're a sugar craver. Watch those sugar cravings lessen once your body starts to enjoy fruit regularly.

Longer-Term Strategy for Better Energy

To improve your energy level over the long term, try the following techniques. Aim to follow this plan for two to three months (imperfectly is fine):

- **Keep caffeine to one to two cups max per day:** Some caffeine can be helpful, but too much can make you extra tired. If you're currently scarfing down coffee just to get through your day, try an experiment. Slowly wean yourself down to two cups max per day and keep it there for two weeks (it takes at least a week to get used to less of a jolt). Assess how you feel after two weeks. If you're like most people, you'll feel more energy without so much caffeine, plus your body will recover faster without all of the stimulants. If you feel nervous about cutting out caffeine too quickly, have as little as you can tolerate. Try a cup of decaf (Swiss Water process is best) if you really like the taste of coffee.

- **Eat lots of cooked veggies:** Cooked veggies are significantly easier on the body, and you can absorb more nutrients from them because their cell walls have been broken during cooking. It's okay to have some raw carrots and a salad or two; just make sure that most of your veggies are cooked. Heap them high on your plate and enjoy!

- **Don't forget about fruit:** Fruit is in the fast energy-boosting category for a reason, but it's good for the long haul, too. Keep up with two to four servings of fruit each day to satisfy your sweet tooth, get loads of vitamins, and get a fast boost of energy.

- **Switch refined sugars for less processed ones:** Trade out white sugar, brown sugar, and high fructose corn syrup for honey, maple syrup, dates, and coconut sugar. These more natural sugars have all of the trace nutrients needed for digestion. The refined sweeteners steal B vitamins and magnesium from your adrenals for digestion, and that theft contributes to low energy.

- **Eat every four to five hours:** For now, try eating something every few hours. You don't have to do this forever, and doing this for the long term might make eating a chore. When you put a large gap between meals, your body uses the stress hormone cortisol to bring blood sugar back up, and right now, a lot of your low energy and fogginess comes from low levels of cortisol, so don't waste this precious hormone this way. Instead, grab a meal or a snack every four hours or so and keep your blood sugar steady.

For many people, an eating schedule might look like this:

- Breakfast at 7:30 a.m.
- Lunch at 12:00 p.m.
- Late afternoon snack at 4:00 p.m.
- Dinner around 6:00 p.m.

If you don't like to eat breakfast, that's okay. Just eat something by 10:00 a.m. to keep your blood sugar steady.

Wrapping It All Up

You'll be surprised how quickly you can start feeling better. When you have even a little bit more energy, it gives you the space to create more health, pleasure, and joy in your life. No matter how tired or burned out you're feeling today, tomorrow can be a better day.

Enjoyment and pleasure can be far down on your to-do list. It also can be challenging to find anything to enjoy in life when your energy is bottomed out. But the pleasurable things in life are what makes living fun, so it's worth improving your energy so you can do things that make you happy.

Finding food pleasurable and enjoyable is a core principle of undieting, and that concept is 100 percent contrary to dieting culture. The dieting culture promotes guilt and shame when it comes to eating, and it's time to let go of those unhelpful and unhealthy ideas.

Pleasure comes back to your life in buckets when your body feels more balanced, your cravings are satisfied, and your diet is balanced for your unique constitution. The best part is that finding deep enjoyment of the food you eat is the best way to understand what your body is looking for. By embracing pure enjoyment in your meals again, you'll find the balanced way of eating your body has been dreaming about.

  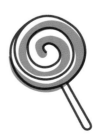

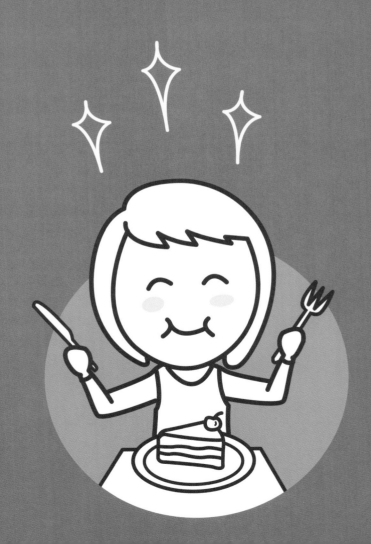

LIVING IN REAL LIFE: MAXIMIZING PLEASURE AND ENJOYMENT

It's one thing to learn and rationally understand what you need to do to create a healthy lifestyle, but it's another challenge to implement it in your real life. It's a challenge that's well worth the effort, though.

By bringing the principles I've talked about throughout this book into your day-to-day practice, you'll gain pleasure, joy, and balance. Your food struggles will be replaced with an inner knowledge of what your body is looking for each day.

If there's one thing I hope you take from this book, it's this: Healthy eating can be pleasurable, and pleasurable eating is much healthier than any diet.

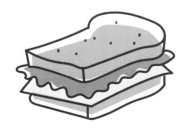

This may seem like a bit of a paradox after years or decades of dieting, but it's true. In fact, it's a cornerstone of the French Paradox, the name for the observation that even though people in France eat a diet that includes a lot of butter, cheese, wine, and bread, they tend to be healthier than people in North America. Why they're healthier has baffled researchers for decades. Some researchers have pointed to the antioxidants in red wine or their use of olive oil rather than inflammatory vegetable oil as what's protecting their hearts from the less favorable aspects of the diet. Others have pointed out that the French diet is a version of The Mediterranean Diet, which has been found to be very healthy (and full of whole food). Although there are many possible reasons why the French lifestyle is so paradoxical, it's the connection to pleasure that's believed to play an important role. Pleasure is a hard thing to quantify and research, but there seems to be a connection. By eating each meal slowly and with enjoyment (instead of guilt), the French people are healthier than their counterparts in other places.

When it comes to maintaining a healthy weight, the United States is ranked as one of the unhealthiest countries in the world, but the population of France is considerably healthier, despite having a diet that historically would have been perceived as unhealthy. I feel there's a lot to be learned from the French way of eating, and attitude might be a factor, as Paul Rozin and his colleagues identified in their research from 1999:

> The group associating food most with health and least with pleasure was the Americans, and the group most pleasure-oriented and least health-oriented was the French. Ironically, the Americans, who make the greatest efforts to alter their diet for the sake of health, are the least likely to classify themselves as healthy eaters.

In France, the quality of the average diet is higher than in the United States, even though each group spends about the same amount of preparation time in the kitchen. The big difference between the two groups occurs at the dinner table. The French spend twice as much time eating and enjoying their food as Americans do. The slow, pleasurable meals the French enjoy automatically manages their portion sizes.

When you eat slowly, your body gets a say in how much you eat. Many people in North America are fast eaters who wolf down their meals in five or ten minutes flat. However, your stomach can take fifteen to twenty minutes to tell your brain that you're full, which means fast eaters may eat much more than necessary before their brains realize it. I firmly believe that it's almost impossible to overeat when you eat slowly; your body just won't let you. You'll feel full long before you've overeaten, and you'll probably be pretty bored before too long.

In North America, people also tend to eat in a distracted way—in front of the TV, in the car, at a desk during work—and this leads to both overeating and a lack of enjoyment of what's being eaten. It may seem counterintuitive, but slow, pleasurable eating helps people eat considerably less at each meal. It's time to be more like the French by reconnecting with the pleasure of meals and enjoying what food brings to your life. Relishing every bite is undieting at its best. Your body is craving something wonderful in this stressful world, and each meal is an opportunity for enjoyment. This is the art of eating and undieting.

Undieting: Relearning the Art of Eating

▌ Take a deep breath, close your eyes, and think about how much you enjoy food.

Consider the following things:

- How often do you savor your meals?
- How often does guilt creep in?
- Do you ever tell yourself, "I shouldn't eat this"?
- Do you think about calories? Or grams of carbs?
- Do you ever punish yourself for indulging in a treat?
- Do you like the flavors and textures of the food you eat?
- Do you worry you might like food a little too much?
- Do you eat food you don't like because it's "healthy"?

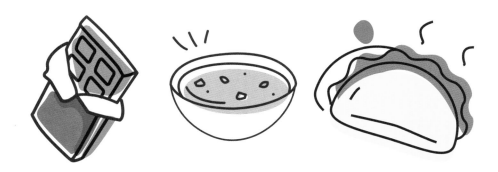

Eating with pleasure and enjoyment can be a struggle for your rational brain, which likes to count calories and judge the quality or quantity of your meals. You may need some time to quiet the obnoxious inner voice that may have been helpful in the past but now tries to keep you inside a dieting regime. Be patient; it takes time to reprogram your rational brain, especially when food manufacturers spend millions of dollars to make their food as addictive as possible. The catchphrase "Betcha can't eat just one!" has a lot of truth in it.

So, how do you, a mere mortal, release yourself from years or decades of counting and judging and steer away from all of the companies trying to compete for space in your kitchen and stomach? The best way I've found to move away from dieting and into pleasure is through a practice I call *conscious eating*.

THE POWER OF CONSCIOUS EATING

The way you eat today is a learned behavior, and at any time, you can learn a new eating behavior. All new habits can be hard to master, and eating habits are particularly difficult to change, so please keep an attitude of kindness for yourself and curiosity throughout this process.

Anytime you eat a meal consciously, you must stay curious. What did you enjoy about the meal? What flavors stood out? Which foods were you most drawn to? What didn't you enjoy about the meal? After you've eaten, consider your energy, your digestion, and how you feel overall. Connect what you ate with how you feel.

When you forget your new habits and let yourself slip into old habits (which will happen), be curious about that too. What was happening on that day that led you to eat a less-than-stellar meal? How did you feel while eating it? What did you feel when you checked in with your body after the meal? How were your energy, your digestion, and your overall well-being?

Conscious eating is a simple habit that pays dividends. When you do it, you automatically exercise portion control because it's challenging to overeat consciously. By paying attention to the food you're eating, you quickly notice the feeling of fullness. Plus, you get a chance to enjoy the food you're having.

The best part is that you automatically shift your diet toward whole food because whole food tastes better when it's chewed and relished. Processed food loses flavor after a couple of chews and generally doesn't taste as good when you pay close attention to the experience of eating it.

Most importantly, conscious eating stops unconscious munching. Every person I've worked with who has tried this technique has discovered an eating habit they weren't aware of, such as absent-mindedly eating food off of their kid's plate or nibbling the food off the cutting board while preparing dinner. One client discovered that she had a habit of eating straight out of her chest freezer, something she had no idea she was doing!

PRACTICING CONSCIOUS EATING

To practice conscious eating, all you need to do is ask yourself two simple yes/no questions:

- Do I want to eat this?

- Do I want to change what I'm doing so I can sit down and enjoy this?

These questions are surprisingly powerful because they take willpower out of the mix entirely. By saying yes in response to both of these questions, you consciously make a choice, and all you need is a quiet spot to practice thorough enjoyment of what you've chosen. When you say no to either question, you make a choice to keep doing whatever you've been doing instead of eating something. This *no* is powerful because it whisks away any longing or wanting while requiring zero willpower because you've actively chosen to forgo the food. You can change your mind at any time.

When you follow a diet, you need to say no to a lot of food during the day. The cookies brought in by a coworker, the lineup of fast-food restaurants on the road home from work when you're *starving*, and any number of other things you "shouldn't" have. Having to decline food repeatedly can nag at you, and those things sit on your shoulder as a reminder that just a few steps away, there's something yummy that you "can't" eat. You can feel deprived, which is a feeling that makes changing habits an almost impossible task. Whenever you feel deprived, you have a deep desire to make that deprivation go away by eating the "forbidden" food. Saying no becomes much more difficult if that voice in your head is saying, "But I *deserve* this!"

With conscious eating, you choose between two options. You never have to pass up something you really want. At any point, you can eat what you desire; you just have to change what you're doing so you can enjoy that food. It's 100 percent your choice. It may seem like this small change in how you say no might not make a big difference, but it *really* does. The freedom of being able to say yes at any time is where the power lies.

With conscious eating, you can eat anything you'd like; you just need to eat your chosen food mindfully. Do you love an evening snack in front of the TV? No problem! You can have that snack or the healthiest alternative, but you need to enjoy it at the kitchen table instead of in the living room. Instead of mindlessly eating a full bag of chips or a full bag of cookies, you'll eat just enough to satisfy your craving. How can you be sure you won't finish off the bag? Simple! You'll want to get back to your TV show!

The process of conscious eating can bring emotional eating to the surface as well. Lots of mindless eating is caused by physical cravings mixed with mindless consumption, but sometimes eating is purely emotional. Food can be a great pacifier, and mindless eating allows you to use food to stuff down your emotions. Conscious eating stops the stuffing down of feelings, which can be powerful and scary. However, you can get a clearer look at those buried emotions so you can deal with them, but, please, reach out for support from a trained counselor or therapist to help process them.

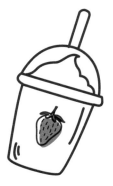

UNCOVERING CHILDHOOD HABITS THAT NO LONGER SERVE YOU

You learn your eating habits as a child, and the habits follow you throughout your life. These habits you learned from your parents helped them get through a meal, but those habits may not be helping you today.

One particular habit—clean your plate—can cause a lot of issues. That habit taught you to override your body's cue of fullness by instead paying attention to the food left on your plate to determine whether the meal is done. I've worked with hundreds of adults who have little sense of feeling full because they've always cleaned their plates. This is a hard habit to release, but it *is* possible.

Slow, mindful eating makes it difficult to eat past the full mark, and, at least at first, putting less food on your plate (knowing that there are second helpings) can help you tap into that full feeling. Changing this habit needs some patience, but you *can* release it.

Keep an eye out for any deeply ingrained habits that might not be serving you anymore. They could include speedy eating, constant snacking, or rewarding yourself with food. Take a hard look; your body wants to release these old habits, and uncovering them is the foundation of making the change.

Releasing Guilt and Shame Over Food Choices

The fastest way to release guilt and shame when you reach for a food you've dubbed as "bad" is by thoroughly enjoying it. Guilt and pleasure can't exist together; this is why permitting yourself to enjoy your favorite food works so brilliantly. Releasing the guilt and shame can be easier said than done, so let's unpack this a bit to help your rational brain get on board.

Decades of dieting culture have conditioned people to judge food as good or bad, and this can make the guilt you might feel when you want to eat something in the "bad" category seem like a normal feeling. Food guilt isn't inherent, though; you've been conditioned to feel it. Food manufacturers can use these conditioned feelings as great drivers to sell you "guilt-free" snacks (remember the commercials for nonfat cookies in the 1980s and '90s?). However, because you've learned to feel a certain way about food, you also can unlearn those feelings.

Guilty feelings block feelings of pleasure, and they also can block any feeling of being satisfied after eating the food that has caused the guilty feelings. The lack of satisfaction can cause you to crave the food even more.

Practicing conscious eating can combat this unpleasant cycle. When you carefully choose to eat a particular food, the next step is simple: Sit down and enjoy the food.

There's power in the simplicity of this. By chewing, tasting, and enjoying the food, your body is getting more than a sense of satiety. Your body knows it's being heard and understood; it also gets to enjoy that wonderful feeling of pleasure.

Remember, some food cravings aren't driven by your body wanting or needing certain nutrients; they're driven by a deep need for pleasure. In your busy life, pleasure is something that you might easily miss. It's not something you can schedule, and it's easy to overlook taking time for pleasure when your to-do list is lengthy. However, although your brain forgets to do pleasurable things, your body doesn't forget, and it might demand a moment of pleasure. Through enjoyment, you give your body something more valuable than nutrients. A pleasurable moment brings you presence and pulls you out of a stressful moment. And at that moment, you also find some joy.

"

Recently, my colleague Carol Domanko reached out to me to share how much undieting has changed her life. Carol, a yoga instructor from Kelowna, British Columbia, has been trapped inside typical dieting culture since she was a preteen. Now in her thirties, Carol's found new freedom in her relationship with food: *I think I started dieting around age eleven or twelve, and instead of becoming healthier, I developed bulimia/anorexia, which I battled until I was in my twenties. It was only when I started "undieting" that I made peace with my body and actually maintained a healthy weight. I've lost 20 pounds in the last year, and it's been effortless keeping it off. I still eat like a queen and don't feel like I need to exercise like a maniac to make up for "cheat days." I just listen to my body and eat real food. It's so simple!*

"

Wrapping It All Up: Embracing Undieting Forever

You show your body deep respect when you tap into its language and *listen*. By not stuffing your body into the teeny tiny box of a strict diet, you give yourself a chance to embrace pleasure again. Every meal can bring your body the nutrients it needs to function correctly, and it can bring pleasure. Pleasure is a cornerstone of a life enjoyed.

By consciously listening to your body and letting it inform you how to eat, you'll have no more counting, depriving, and stressing about what's good or bad. Instead, you just get to enjoy food—whole food, whole ingredients, whole enjoyment.

To live a life of undieting forever, work on making the following concepts your new habits so that you can shed the old, unhelpful habits:

AVOID NUTRITIONAL FASHIONS

Any nutritional expert, book, or recommendation that lists one macronutrient as "bad" and another as "good" is the hallmark of a fad diet. Avoid these at all costs. Remember that there aren't any nutrient villains or heroes, and you shouldn't have to count calories or macros to give your body healthy, balanced meals.

I can guarantee that any new diet that comes along and is highly recommended will go out of style as quickly as the hottest new shoe on the market. Whoever might be promoting the diets will also usually try to convince you that they've finally found the answer—the perfect answer for everyone for all time. But, very soon, the recommendation will be as relevant as a pair of bright orange leg warmers from the 1980s. It's your body that has the real answer. Tap into that.

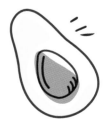

CONNECT TO YOUR BODY'S NEEDS AND WANTS THROUGH YOUR CRAVINGS

One of the fastest ways to understand what your body is looking for is by listening to your cravings. Your body is looking for vitamins, minerals, nutrients, pleasure, and a whole host of components that scientists haven't uncovered yet. Your body knows what you need, and by listening to and respecting your cravings, you can show your body that you care. Paying attention to your body is excellent self-care.

Your rational brain may fight back against some cravings, such as for candy or cake, but trust in the wisdom of your body. What might it be looking for? Is there a way to satisfy the craving with whole food?

A healthy diet doesn't need to be a "perfect" one. Although it's not a formally recognized condition, orthorexia is a growing concern. Those dealing with orthorexia are obsessed with eating a perfect diet, and that obsession outweighs the enjoyment of eating. I've worked with quite a few people with many symptoms of orthorexia, and I've noticed an interesting truth: What most health experts would deem an absolutely "perfect" diet is actually an unhealthy one. In my experience, those people with symptoms of orthorexia still suffer from many health issues that we often associate with highly processed diets. I also believe that the rise of more extreme fad diets is triggering more and more people into an orthorexic state.

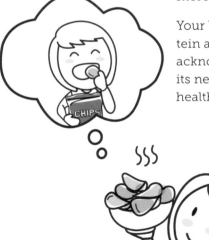

Your body needs to enjoy your food, just like it needs protein and magnesium. By listening to your body's quiet voice, acknowledging what it's looking for, and trying to understand its needs, you're taking a powerful step to creating a happy, healthy, and balanced body.

LISTEN TO YOUR DIGESTIVE SYSTEM'S WISDOM AND OPTIMIZE YOUR ASSIMILATION

Through the enteric nervous system (ENS) that surrounds your digestive organs, your gut sends your brain much more information than your brain sends your gut. Through a complex cocktail of neurotransmitters, immune cells, and gut bacteria, you can glean a lot of information about how your body is doing by listening to your gut.

The gut is the place where all of your food is broken down, absorbed, and assimilated, so your body can use the nutrients to create muscles, bones, hormones, and every cell in your body. The ecosystem of bacteria in your small and large intestines plays a powerful role in digestion and also balances your immune system, modulates inflammation, stokes metabolism, and may play a role in mood and even personality.

Listen to your digestive symptoms, even the quiet and easily ignored ones like a bit of gas, and you'll be able to optimize your digestion and assimilation processes. Be kind to your gut, and your whole body will sing!

FIND BALANCE IN THIS STRESSFUL WORLD AND BRING YOUR ENERGY BACK

It may seem almost impossible to find some time to relax each day within your busy life. As a society, we've come to idolize busy-ness, and our social media feeds are full of tips and tricks to get more done in a day. People are trying to hack their lives instead of being inside their lives.

Taking a few deep breaths, enjoying a moment of presence with your kids or pets, and walking in the park are beautiful ways to move out of the high-stress/high-cortisol reality of your days and into a balanced, rejuvenating relaxed state. Every single moment counts. Don't underestimate the power of just a moment of presence. They all add up to a happier, more balanced body.

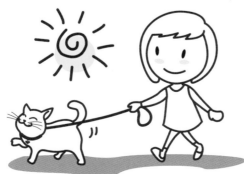

RETURN TO PLEASURE AND JOY THROUGH CONSCIOUS EATING

Cravings for pleasure can feel counterintuitive, and they're the most common cravings that people deprive themselves of when they're shifting to a whole food–based way of eating. By consciously choosing to enjoy some of the foods you crave—and I mean *really* enjoying them—then you can satisfy your craving quickly. Over time, denying these cravings can result in guilt-ridden food binges. Consciously enjoying all food will melt guilt away quickly and bring your body what it was looking for: pleasure.

Eat slowly and chew well to manage how much you eat at each meal. When you eat quickly and distractedly, you tend to eat way more than you need to eat. The practice of conscious eating is one of the powerful ways to balance weight, reduce digestive symptoms, and simply enjoy life a wee bit more. It's a practice that fully respects your body.

EMBRACE YOUR BODY'S WISDOM THROUGH UNDIETING

No matter where you are right now in your health journey, you're just one small change away from more energy, a clearer mind, and a healthier body. One small change, one that you're 95 percent confident that you can knock out of the park, is all it takes. It's a great way to start a whole new healthy life.

I feel so inspired and humbled every time I watch someone transform from a dieting mentality to undieting. It's a magical moment to watch them tap into their body's wisdom and understand how to feed their body. There's so much freedom to be felt in that moment; never again will they question whether a new hot diet is for them. Instead, they know deep down that following any fad diet is counter to what they know. In short, they know their body.

You already have plenty of stresses in your life, and figuring out what to eat doesn't need to be one of them. By shifting to a whole-food diet that's balanced for your unique constitution, you can get off the stressful roller coaster of dieting and food guilt and replace negative feelings with sheer food pleasure.

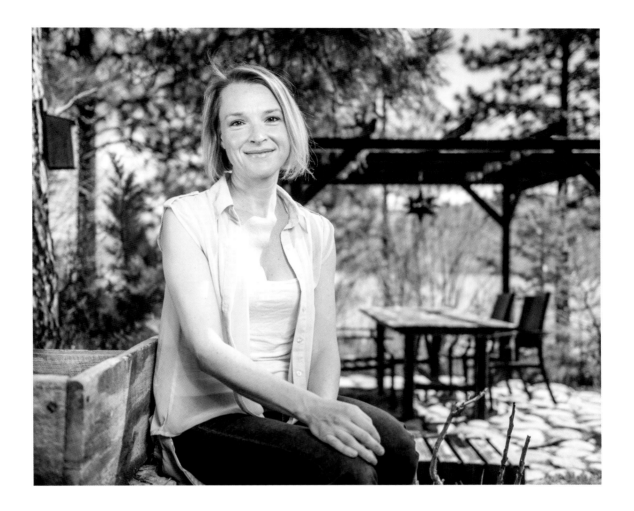

By tuning into your body's needs and wants, you can glide into a healthy diet without using any willpower and without feeling deprived. Instead, each day your diet adds a little bit more pleasure and joy to your life.

You are already a nutrition expert, so get off the fad dieting treadmill and into *undieting.* It's healthy eating at its best.

NUTRITIÓNIST

Lisa Kilgour

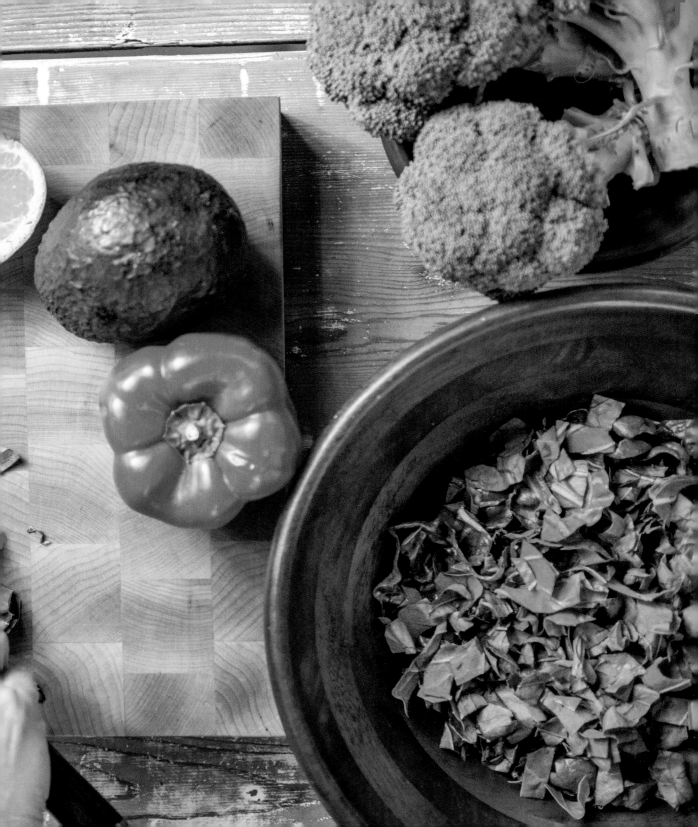

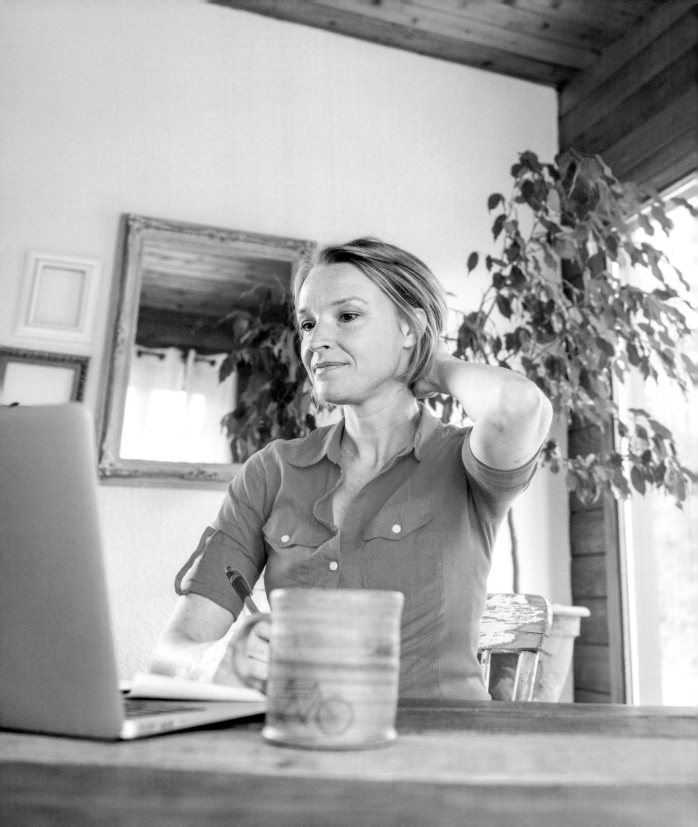

REFERENCES

CHAPTER 1

Brown University. "Gut Microbiome Regulates the Intestinal Immune System." ScienceDaily website, December 18, 2018, https://www.sciencedaily.com/releases/2018/12/181218123123.htm.

M. Cohut. "How Diet Can Alter the Gut, Leading to Insulin Resistance." Medical News Today website, August 15, 2019, https://www.medicalnewstoday.com/articles/326050.

J. DiNicolantonio. "The Cardiometabolic Consequences of Replacing Saturated Fats with Carbohydrates or Ω-6 Polyunsaturated Fats: Do the Dietary Guidelines Have It Wrong?" *Open Heart* 1, no. 1 (2014). doi:10.1136/openhrt-2013-000032.

C. Gardner et al. "Effect of Low-Fat vs Low-Carbohydrate Diet on 12-Month Weight Loss in Overweight Adults and the Association with Genotype Pattern or Insulin Secretion." *JAMA* 319, no. 7 (2018): 667–679. doi:10.1001/jama.2018.0245.

K. Gunnars. "Do Low-Fat Diets Really Work?" Healthline website, March 27, 2018, https://www.healthline.com/nutrition/do-low-fat-diets-work.

A. Hakansson and G. Molin. "Gut Microbiota and Inflammation." *Nutrients* 3, no. 6 (2011): 637–682. doi:10.3390/nu3060637.

P. Hernández-Alonso et al. "High Dietary Protein Intake Is Associated with an Increased Body Weight and Total Death Risk." *Clinical Nutrition* 35, no. 2 (2016): 496–506. doi:10.1016/j.clnu.2015.03.016.

Y. Hewlings-Martin. "Loss of Microbial Gut Diversity a Threat to Health?" Medical News Today website, August 27, 2017, https://www.medicalnewstoday.com/articles/319161.

P. M. Kris-Etherton et al. "Polyunsaturated Fatty Acids in the Food Chain in the United States." *The American Journal of Clinical Nutrition* 71, no. 1 (2000): 179S–188S. doi:10.1093/ajcn/71.1.179S.

Lund University. "New Link Between Gut Bacteria and Obesity." ScienceDaily website, February 23, 2018, https://www.sciencedaily.com/releases/2018/02/180223092441.htm.

P. Martyn-Nemeth, L. Quinn, U. Menon, S. Shrestha, C. Pate, and G. Shah. "Dietary Profiles of First-Generation South Asian Indian Adolescents in the United States." *Journal of Immigrant and Minority Health* 19, no. 2 (2017): 309–317. doi:10.1007/s10903-016-0382-6.

C. Masterjohn. "Saturated Fat Does a Body Good." The Weston A. Price Foundation website, May 6, 2016, https://www.westonaprice.org/health-topics/abcs-of-nutrition/saturated-fat-body-good/.

P. W. Parodi. "Conjugated Linoleic Acid and Other Anticarcinogenic Agents of Bovine Milk Fat." *Journal of Dairy Science* 82, no. 6 (1999): 1339–1349. doi:10.3168/jds.S0022-0302(99)75358-0.

J. Reedy. "How the U.S. Low-Fat Diet Recommendations of 1977 Contributed to the Declining Health of Americans." (honors scholar thesis, University of Connecticut, 2016), https://opencommons.uconn.edu/cgi/viewcontent.cgi?article=1482&context=srhonors_theses.

D. Robson. "A High-Carb Diet May Explain Why Okinawans Live So Long." BBC Future website, January 17, 2019, https://www.bbc.com/future/article/20190116-a-high-carb-diet-may-explain-why-okinawans-live-so-long.

B. St. Pierre. "Carb Controversy: Why Low-Carb Diets Have It All Wrong." Precision Nutrition website, https://www.precisionnutrition.com/low-carb-diets.

CHAPTER 2

M. Pollan. *In Defense of Food*. (New York: Penguin Press, 2009).

P. W. Siri-Tarino, Q. Sun, F. B. Hu, and R. M. Krauss. "Meta-Analysis of Prospective Cohort Studies Evaluating the Association of Saturated Fat with Cardiovascular Disease." *The American Journal of Clinical Nutrition* 91, no. 3 (2010): 535–546. doi:10.3945/ajcn.2009.27725.

CHAPTER 3

M. A. Cheeseman. "Artificial Food Color Additives and Child Behavior." *Environmental Health Perspectives* 120, no. 1 (2012): a15–a16. doi:10.1289/ehp.1104409.

J. Firger. "Food Additives Linked to Obesity, Digestive Problems in Study." CBS News website, February 25, 2015, https://www.cbsnews.com/news/food-additives-linked-to-obesity-digestive-problems/.

P. Jakszyn and C. A. Gonzalez. "Nitrosamine and Related Food Intake and Gastric and Oesophageal Cancer Risk: A Systematic Review of the Epidemiological Evidence." *World Journal of Gastroenterology* 12, no. 27 (2006): 4296–4303. doi:10.3748/wjg.v12.i27.4296.

R. Tippet. "Mortality and Cause of Death, 1900 v. 2010." Carolina Demography website, June 16, 2014, https://www.ncdemography.org/2014/06/16/mortality-and-cause-of-death-1900-v-2010/.

CHAPTER 4

C. Domonoske. "50 Years Ago, Sugar Industry Quietly Paid Scientists to Point Blame at Fat." NPR website, September 13, 2016, https://www.npr.org/sections/thetwo-way/2016/09/13/493739074/50-years-ago-sugar-industry-quietly-paid-scientists-to-point-blame-at-fat.

C. E. Kearns, L. A. Schmidt, and S. A. Glantz. "Sugar Industry and Coronary Heart Disease Research: A Historical Analysis of Internal Industry Documents." *JAMA Internal Medicine* 176, no. 11 (2016): 1680–1685. doi:10.1001/jamainternmed.2016.5394.

A. O'Connor. "How the Sugar Industry Shifted Blame to Fat." *New York Times,* September 12, 2016, https://www.nytimes.com/2016/09/13/well/eat/how-the-sugar-industry-shifted-blame-to-fat.html?action=click&contentCollection=Opinion&module=Trending&version=Full&region=Marginalia&pgtype=article.

CHAPTER 5

F. J. Clemente et al. "A Selective Sweep on a Deleterious Mutation in CPT1A in Arctic Populations." *American Journal of Human Genetics* 95, no. 5 (2014): 584–589. doi:10.1016/j.ajhg.2014.09.016.

L. Cornaro. *The Art of Living Long.* (Whitefish, MT: Kessinger Publishing, 2010).

L. Foxcroft. "Lord Byron: The Celebrity Diet Icon." BBC News Magazine, January 3, 2012, https://www.bbc.com/news/magazine-16351761.

F. Spritzler. "Do 'Diets' Really Just Make You Fatter?" Healthline website, March 9, 2020, https://www.healthline.com/nutrition/do-diets-make-you-gain-weight#section2.

CHAPTER 6

C. D. Davis. "The Gut Microbiome and Its Role in Obesity." *Nutrition Today* 51, no. 4 (2016): 167–174. doi:10.1097/NT.0000000000000167.

Cleveland Clinic. "Why People Diet, Lose Weight and Gain It All Back." Health Essentials website, October 1, 2019, https://health.clevelandclinic.org/why-people-diet-lose-weight-and-gain-it-all-back/.

K. M. Flegal, B. K. Kit, and H. Orpana. "Association of All-Cause Mortality with Overweight and Obesity Using Standard Body Mass Index Categories: A Systematic Review and Meta-Analysis." *JAMA* 309, no. 1 (2013): 71–82. doi:10.1001/jama.2012.113905.

E. Fothergill et al. "Persistent Metabolic Adaptation 6 Years after 'The Biggest Loser' Competition." *Obesity* 24, no. 8 (2016): 1612–1619. doi:10.1002/oby.21538.

T. D. Freuman. "When Nutrition Labels Lie." U.S. News & World Report website, August 21, 2012, https://health.usnews.com/health-news/blogs/eat-run/2012/08/21/when-nutrition-labels-lie.

D. Grady. "The Fit Tend to Fidget, and Biology May Be Why, a Study Says." *New York Times,* January 28, 2005, https://www.nytimes.com/2005/01/28/health/the-fit-tend-to-fidget-and-biology-may-be-why-a-study-says.html.

J. E. Oliver. *Fat Politics: The Real Story Behind America's Obesity Epidemic* (New York: Oxford University Press, 2006).

L. M. Redman and E. Ravussin. "Caloric Restriction in Humans: Impact on Physiological, Psychological, and Behavioral Outcomes." *Antioxidants & Redox Signaling* 14, no. 2 (2011): 275–287. doi:10.1089/ars.2010.3253.

Rowett Research Institute. "Very Low Carbohydrate Diets May Disrupt Long-Term Gut Health." ScienceDaily website, June 20, 2007, https://www.sciencedaily.com/releases/2007/06/070619173537.htm.

University of California – Los Angeles. "Dieting Does Not Work, Researchers Report." ScienceDaily website, April 5, 2007, https://www.sciencedaily.com/releases/2007/04/070404162428.htm.

University of California – San Diego. "Big Data from World's Largest Citizen Science Microbiome Project Serves Food for Thought." ScienceDaily website, May 15, 2018, https://www.sciencedaily.com/releases/2018/05/180515092931.htm.

CHAPTER 8

J. Allen, interview by Guy Raz, *All Things Considered,* NPR, June 2, 2012, https://www.npr.org/2012/06/02/154212561/why-do-humans-crave-crispy-food.

K. Bruinsma and D. L. Taren. "Chocolate: Food or Drug?" *Journal of the American Dietetic Association* 99, no. 10 (1999): 1249–1256. doi:10.1016/S0002-8223(99)00307-7.

E. Deans. "Sunlight, Sugar, and Serotonin." Psychology Today website, May 9, 2011, https://www.psychologytoday.com/ca/blog/evolutionary-psychiatry/201105/sunlight-sugar-and-serotonin.

E. Donga. "A Single Night of Partial Sleep Deprivation Induces Insulin Resistance in Multiple Metabolic Pathways in Healthy Subjects." *Journal of Clinical Endocrinology and Metabolism* 95, no. 6 (2010): 2963–2968. doi:10.1210/jc.2009-2430.

J. K. Kiecolt-Glaser. "Stress, Food, and Inflammation: Psychoneuroimmunology and Nutrition at the Cutting Edge." *Psychosomatic Medicine* 72, no. 4 (2010): 365–369. doi:10.1097/PSY.0b013e3181dbf489.

A. Mente et al. "Urinary Sodium Excretion, Blood Pressure, Cardiovascular Disease, and Mortality: A Community-Level Prospective Epidemiological Cohort Study." *The Lancet* 392, no. 10146 (2018): 496–506. doi:10.1016/S0140-6736(18)31376-X.

O. Mesarwi, J. Polak, J. Jun, and V. Y. Polotsky. "Sleep Disorders and the Development of Insulin Resistance and Obesity." *Endocrinology & Metabolism Clinics of North America* 42, no. 3 (2013): 617–634. doi:10.1016/j.ecl.2013.05.001.

T. Newman. "High Blood Pressure: Sodium May Not Be the Culprit." MedicalNewsToday website, April 25, 2017, https://www.medicalnewstoday.com/articles/317099.php#5.

M. Schatzker. *The Dorito Effect* (New York: Simon & Schuster, 2016).

S. Yanovski. "Sugar and Fat: Cravings and Aversions." *The Journal of Nutrition* 133, no. 3 (2003): 835S–837S. doi:10.1093/jn/133.3.835S.

CHAPTER 9

A. Abbott. "Scientists Bust Myth That Our Bodies Have More Bacteria Than Human Cells." Nature website, January 8, 2016, https://www.nature.com/news/scientists-bust-myth-that-our-bodies-have-more-bacteria-than-human-cells-1.19136.

American Academy of Pediatrics. "The History of Antibiotics." HealthyChildren.org website, updated November 15, 2019, https://www.healthychildren.org/English/health-issues/conditions/treatments/Pages/The-History-of-Antibiotics.aspx.

Y. Belkaid and T. Hand. "Role of the Microbiota in Immunity and Inflammation." *Cell* 152, no. 1 (2014): 121–141. doi:10.1016/j.cell.2014.03.011.

P. Bercik et al. "The Intestinal Microbiota Affect Central Levels of Brain-Derived Neurotrophic Factor and Behavior in Mice." *Gastroentrology* 141, no. 2 (2011): 599–609. doi:10.1053/j.gastro.2011.04.052.

M. Blaser, interview by Terry Gross, *Fresh Air,* NPR, April 14, 2014, https://www.npr.org/2014/04/14/302899093/modern-medicine-may-not-be-doing-your-microbiome-any-favors.

T. W. Buford. "(Dis)Trust Your Gut: The Gut Microbiome in Age-Related Inflammation, Health, and Disease." *Microbiome* 5 (2017): 80. doi:10.1186/s40168-017-0296-0.

L. M. Christian et al. "Gut Microbiome Composition Is Associated with Temperament During Early Childhood." *Brain, Behavior, and Immunity* 45 (2015): 118. doi:10.1016/j.bbi.2014.10.018.

M. Fadgyas-Stanculete, A-M. Buga, A. Popa-Wagner, and D. L. Dumitrascu. "The Relationship Between Irritable Bowel Syndrome and Psychiatric Disorders: From Molecular Changes to Clinical Manifestations." *Journal of Molecular Psychiatry* 2, no. 1 (2014): 4. doi:10.1186/2049-9256-2-4.

A. Kondrashov et al. "A Six-Fold Gradient in the Incidence of Type 1 Diabetes at the Eastern Border of Finland." *Annals of Medicine* 37, no. 1 (2005): 67–72. doi:10.1080/07853890410018952.

B. Li, C. Selmi, R. Tang, M. E. Gershwin, and X. Ma. "The Microbiome and Autoimmunity: A Paradigm from the Gut-Liver Axis." *Cellular & Molecular Immunology* 15 (2018): 595–609. doi:10.1038/cmi.2018.7.

P. Luczynski et al. "Growing Up in a Bubble: Using Germ-Free Animals to Assess the Influence of the Gut Microbiota on Brain and Behavior." *International Journal of Neuropsychopharmacology* 19, no. 8 (2016): pyw020. doi:10.1093/ijnp/pyw020.

T. Ramatla, L. Ngoma, M. Adetunji, and M. Mwanza. "Evaluation of Antibiotic Residues in Raw Meat Using Different Analytical Methods." *Antibiotics (Basel)* 6, no. 4 (2017): 34. doi:10.3390/antibiotics6040034.

B. Stockton, and M. Davies. "Antibiotic Use Plummets on US Farms After Ban on Using Drugs to Make Livestock Grow Faster." The Bureau of Investigative Journalism website, December 19, 2018, https://www.thebureauinvestigates.com/stories/2018-12-19/antibiotic-use-falls-on-us-farms-after-ban-on-using-drugs-to-make-livestock-grow-faster.

CHAPTER 10

World Health Organization. "Burn-Out an 'Occupational Phenomenon': International Classification of Diseases." World Health Organization website, May 28, 2019, https://www.who.int/mental_health/evidence/burn-out/en.

CHAPTER 11

Independent Media Institute. "Food Companies Are Making Their Products Addictive, and It's Sickening (Literally)," EcoWatch website, March 26, 2019, https://www.ecowatch.com/food-companies-making-products-addictive-2632845184.html.

National Eating Disorders Association. Orthorexia definition, NEDA website, https://www.nationaleatingdisorders.org/learn/by-eating-disorder/other/orthorexia.

M. Oaklander. "8 Secrets to Eating Like a French Person," Time website, June 30, 2016, https://time.com/4389492/french-person-diet-cheese-wine/.

L. H. Powell, C. Shima, R. Kazlauskaite, and B. M. Appelhans. "Lifestyle in France and the United States: An American Perspective." *Journal of the American Dietetic Association* 110, no. 6 (2010): 845–847. doi:10.1016/j.jada.2010.03.029.

M. Rao and M. D. Gershon. "The Bowel and Beyond: The Enteric Nervous System in Neurological Disorders." *Nature Reviews Gastroenterology & Hepatology* 13, no. 9 (2016): 517–528. doi:10.1038/nrgastro.2016.107.

P. Rozin, C. Fischler, S. Imada, A. Sarubin, and A. Wrzesniewski. "Attitudes to Food and the Role of Food in Life in the USA, Japan, Flemish Belgium and France: Possible Implications for the Diet–Health Debate." *Appetite* 33, no. 2 (1999): 163–180. doi:10.1006/appe.1999.0244.

C. O. C. Werle, B. Wansink, and C. R. Payne. "Is It Fun or Exercise? The Framing of Physical Activity Biases Subsequent Snacking." *Marketing Letters* 26 (2015): 691–702. doi:10.1007/s11002-014-9301-6.

F. Whittaker-Wood. "New Map: The Most Unhealthy Countries in the World." Clinic Compare website, September 22, 2017, https://blog.cliniccompare.co.uk/most-unhealthy-countries.

ACKNOWLEDGMENTS

Thank you so much for reading this book all the way to the end. I'm so grateful to you for spending this time reading my words. Without you, there's no reason to write. Thank you.

To everyone I've worked with closely as a nutritionist, thank you for your openness and for sharing your story with me. Every single one of you helped me grow as a practitioner, and you've helped me see the power of undieting in real life. Thank you.

A big BIG thank you to my partner Michael. You not only put up with my crazy writing mode for months but you also read each and every word, fixing a lot of my troubling grammar, and you gave me very thoughtful ideas and recommendations that made this book so much better. Thank you, Love.

To Julie, my longtime friend and source of inspiration, who showed me that finishing a giant bear of a project is possible. Every time I got stuck or felt like there's no way I can finish, I remembered that this book is tiny compared to a PhD dissertation, and if you can rock your diss, I can finish this book. Thank you for showing me what's possible.

To Nicole, my friend and cheerleader. Thank you for having my back, for giving me so many great ideas, and for pushing me through so many hurdles. Much of my work has been inspired by you.

To Susan and Diana, my friends, guides, and mentors. Thank you in every way for helping me get to where I am today. I'm the person I am today because of both of you. Thank you.

To Charlotte, my brilliant editor. Thank you for clearing through all of the muck and making my message clear. You really got me and what I was trying to say, and you made the editing process (almost) easy. Thank you.

To Stephanie, who "found" me. Thank you for that glorious email in the fall of 2019 that asked a possibly life-changing question, "Would you like to write a book about undieting?" Little did you know that you had read my mind and that this was a book that had been percolating in my head for many months. Thank you for making this idea come to life.

To everyone at Fremont Press, thank you for taking a chance with me, an unknown author, and giving me the opportunity to write about a topic I'm so passionate about. Thank you for all of your support with this book and for teaching me so much about publishing. An extra thank you to Susan Lloyd for all of your support and our great chats.

And lastly, and importantly, to my family. Thank you for supporting me throughout all of the different incarnations in my life and for supporting me even while I live on the other side of the country. I always know that I have a soft place to fall anytime there are wolves at my door. Thank you.

Lisa Kilgour

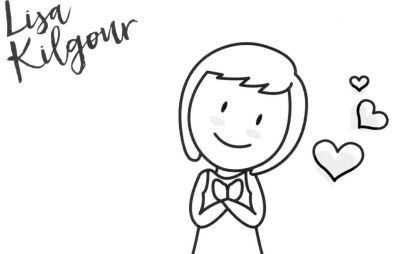

INDEX

enjoyment. *See* pleasure and enjoyment
enteric nervous system (ENS), 132, 138, 169
evening cravings, 127, 128
exhaustion, 147
extra-virgin olive oil, 31

F
fad diets
    in 1900s, 75–76
    about, 73, 82
    Atkins diet, 76–77
    avoiding, 167
    current, 77–79
    hallmarks of, 79–81
    origins of, 74
fat
    in the 1980s, 26–27
    about, 26
    calories in, 26
    as a carrier for nutrients, 27
    healthy, 31
    importance of, 27–28
    lack of nutrients in, 28
    monounsaturated, 28–29
    polyunsaturated, 28–29
    saturated, 28–29
    types of dietary, 28–29
    unsaturated, 28–30
Fat Politics (Oliver), 92
federal dietary guidelines, 68–69
fermented foods, 136, 144
fiber, 54, 140
fish, as a healthy fatty food, 31
flatulence, 137
flax, 143
flaxseed oil, 31
Fletcher, Horace, 75
Fletcherizing, 75
flour, 54
food freedom, 52
food frequency questionnaires, 44
food manufacturers
    about, 42–43, 48, 71
    competing for stomach share, 66
    federal dietary guidelines, 68–69

    influence on dietary recommendations
      by, 67–68
    navigating grocery stores, 69–70
    profit-driven motivations of, 65–71
food repeating, 137
food sensitivities, 137, 141
French Paradox, 159–161
fruit
    for afternoon cravings, 127
    benefits of, 21
    for candy cravings, 118
    as a fast energy booster, 155, 156
    shopping for, 59–60
    for sweet cravings, 115
Funk, Casimir, 41

G
gas, 137, 139
GERD, 137, 141
ghrelin, 80
glucose, 21, 23–24, 77–78
gluten, 104
grains, essential amino acids in, 33
grocery stores, navigating, 69–70
guilt, over food choices, 165–166
gut bacteria, 91, 136, 143–144
gut reset, 142–145
gut/brain connection, 132–133
gut-healing foods, 144–145
gut/immune connection, 134–135

H
hair, protein for, 34
healthy eater bias, 43
healthy fat, 31
heaviness, 137, 141
hemp seed oil, 31
Himalayan salt, 122–123, 128
honey, for candy cravings, 118
hormonal imbalances, 25
hummus, 54
hunger hormone, 80
hypothyroid, 154

ABOUT THE AUTHOR

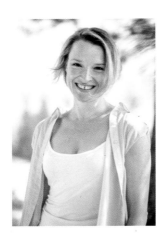

Lisa Kilgour is Certified in Holistic Nutrition and is a sought-after speaker, educator, and writer who specializes in real-life healthy eating.

Refusing to accept a one-size-fits-all approach to nutrition, Lisa teaches the skills that help people uncover their unique health puzzles to find the way of eating that keeps their bodies and minds happy and healthy.

In 2015, Lisa spoke about the gut-brain connection at TEDx Kelowna, and in 2010 she was voted "BC's Favorite Nutritionist" by Natural Care Canada.

Lisa lives with her three rambunctious cats and partner Michael in the breathtaking Okanagan Valley in British Columbia, Canada, where she's surrounded by local, healthy food and stunning scenery.